Chronic Fatigue Syndrome

Chronic Fatigue Syndrome

Edited by

Shlomo Yehuda

Bar Ilan University
Ramat Gan, Israel

and

David I. Mostofsky

Boston University
Boston, Massachusetts

Plenum Press • New York and London

Library of Congress Cataloging-in-Publication Data

On file

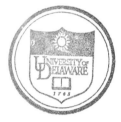

RB
150
.F37
C4733
1997

Proceedings of the Second Farber Center International Conference on Chronic Fatigue Syndrome, held December 12 – 13, 1995, at Bar-Ilan University in Ramat Gan, Israel

ISBN 0-306-45587-0

© 1997 Plenum Press, New York
A Division of Plenum Publishing Corporation
233 Spring Street, New York, N. Y. 10013

http://www.plenum.com

10 9 8 7 6 5 4 3 2 1

Printed in the United States of America

PREFACE

Shlomo Yehuda and David I. Mostofsky

The Second Farber Center International Conference was held on December 19th, 1995 at Bar Ilan University, Israel. The topic of the conference was: "Chronic Fatigue Syndrome." The members of the Scientific Committee were: Prof. Yehuda, Prof. Mostofsky, Mr. Riesenberg, and Prof. Sredni. This conference was supported by the Farber Center for Alzheimer Research, the Ginsburg Chair for Research into Alzheimer Disease, and by the Gold Foundation. The present volume summarizes the controversial and interesting issues as well as the experimental and research results as discussed by the distinguished invited speakers.

The term "chronic fatigue syndrome" was created to describe a group of symptoms that has often been popularly referred to as the "yuppie flu." The unusual and puzzling symptoms of CFS include severe fatigue, weakness, fever, depression, and sore throat and lymph nodes. Several other disorders seem to share many of the CFS's symptoms to various degrees and since no undisputed biological etiology has been identified, it has often been regarded with great suspicion as a legitimate and organic disorder. Only in cases of infectious mononucleosis ("kissing disease") was the Epstein–Barr herpes virus found. The controversy among physicians and other health care professionals concerns the very existence of CFS as a unique

entity well differentiated from other terms such as fibromyalgia, neurasthenia, or special kinds of depression. (For
examples, see: Goldenberg, 1990; Millenson, 1992; Butler
et al, 1991; Cleare et al, 1995; Deluca et al, 1995; White,
1995.)

Among the presenting symptoms, relatively little attention is given to the subjective feeling of the CFS patients, who report that they suffer from a decline in
cognitive functions. While there are few research reports in
the literature, an examination of their findings was not
particularly rewarding and did not allow the development
of a unified or clear understanding. Each article appears to
stand by itself, and comparisons of one study to another
are at best difficult. We recently completed an analysis of
17 papers that have been published on this topic. Several
issues emerged during the analysis attempting to relate
CFS and cognitive functions: (a) there is no single set of diagnostic criteria for CFS; (b) there is no agreement on what
ought to constitute the appropriate control group (indeed
some studies did not include any control group); (c) some
studies included measurements of the levels of depression,
and others do not; (d) different studies used different
neuropsychological tests and measured different cognitive
dimensions; (e) the use of statistical analytic tools differs
from one study to another. These and other problems prevent treatment of data with more sophisticated tools (such
as meta-analysis methods) that might allow an integration
of all the data and permit a statistical basis for assessing
the relative importance of each variable tested in these
studies. One general picture is clear: the patients indeed
suffer from transient cognitive decline. However, it is difficult to compare these studies in order to validate the results on particular aspects of cognition. It is hard to
determine whether CFS *per se* has an effect on cognitive
functions or whether the decline in cognitive function is
the result of depression. The results of our study are summarized in Table 1.

If indeed CSF is related to some malfunction of the immune system, and if the cognitive decline is real and asso-

Table 1.

Reference	N subjects	N (control)	CFS criteria	Statistical tests	Measures
Altay et al., 1990	21	Normative samples matched by age. N not specified; reference not specified.	PIN. Doctors diagnose according to specified criteria. Post hoc analysis showed CDC matched.	t-tests, M ± SD	*Attention impairments-* Trails A&B WAIS-R: digit symbol, similarity test. *Intellectual Functioning-* Shipley Living Scale
Powell et al., 1990	58	33 depressed	Unexplained fatigue; fulfilled Dawson, 1990 criteria for CFS.	Non-parametric tests: χ^2, Kruskal-Wallis ANOVA, χ^2, Wilcoxon.	Self Assessment Questionnaire: attribution of symptoms. Schedule For Affective Disorder and Schizophrenia (SADS).
Butler et al., 1991	50	50 (same subjects before and after).	Sickness period: 5 years.	t-test, χ^2, Wilcoxon.	Beck Depression Inventory, General Health Questionnaire, Hospital Anxiety and Depression Scale
Daugherty et al., 1991	19	Comparison to norms according to age.	Features that contributed to the formation of the CDC criteria.	Average percentage of points below the norm	MMPI, Wisconsin's Neuropsychological Battery Test; IQ, Attention, Sequencing Ability, Problem Solving, Kinesthetic Deficit, Motor Skills, Verbal Memory, Visual Memory.
Lane et al., 1991	60	60 with fatigue complaints.	Criteria specified in the article.	M ± SD, χ^2, t-test.	Diagnostic Interview Schedule of the National Institute of Mental Health (DIS-III-A).
Scheffers et al., 1992	13	13 healthy subjects matched by age, sex education.	CDC criteria	F, M ± SD	WAIS-R Wechsler Memory Scale, Beck Depression Inventory, Modified Spielberger State Anxiety Inventory, Attention Paradigm, Visual Oddball Paradigm, EEG.
Bonner et al., 1993	46	46 (same subjects before and after)	Fatigue questionnaire, general health questionnaire, hospital anxiety and depression questionnaire	χ^2, Mann-Whitney U test.	Interview that used: Schedule for Affective Disorder and Schizophrenia (SADS), Beck Depression Inventory, Modified Somatic Discomfort Questionnaire, Self-Assessment Scale of Functional Impairment, Self Rated Global Improvement.
Deluca et al., 1993	12	11 MS patients.11 healthy subjects, matched by age, education and verbal intelligence.	CDC criteria.	F-tests, Pearson r, M ± SEM	Paced Auditory Serial Addition Test (PASAT). WAIS-R: digit span: vocabulary, similarities. Verbal IQ. Beck depression inventory.

Table 1. *Continued)*

Reference	N subjects	N (control)	CFS criteria	Statistical tests	Measures
Grafman et al., 1993	20	17 healthy, matched by age, education and handedness.	20, first survey respondents. Criteria not specified.	F tests	*Intellectual Functioning*- WAIS-R *Timing and Reaction time (RT)*- Simple RT. Serial RT. Time Wall. Time Clock *Problem solving and Planning*- Tower of London. Tower of Hanoi. General Questions. *Memory*- Wechsler Memory Scale. Paired Association, Hasher Monitoring Task. Story Memory. Word Fluency. *Mood and Physical Condition*- Beck; Somatisation Scale. Neurobehavioral Rating Scale. Fatigue Scale.
McDonald et al., 1993	65	No control group.	Specific criteria and Sharpe et al., 1991 criteria.	M ± SD, %	*Psychiatric interview*- Revised Clinical Interview Schedule (CIS-R), ICD-9 Criteria. Self and Family Report of Psychiatric History. The Social Supports and Stresses Instruments (SSSI).
Ray et al., 1993	24	24 friends or relatives accompanying CFS patients.	Sharpe et al., 1991 criteria.	M ± SD, t-test, Pearson r	Everyday Attention Questionnaire (EAQ). Profile of Fatigue Related Symptoms, Stroop Test, the Embedded Figure Test (EFT).
Smith et al., 1993	57	19 healthy hospital staff.	Criteria specified in article.	F, M ± SD	*Depression*- Middlesex Hospital Questionnaire Revised. Spielberger State Anxiety Inventory. Cohen-Hobermann Index of Physical Symptoms. Cognitive Failures Questionnaire. Mood- Analogue Scale. *Psychomotor tasks*- Simple Reaction Time. Choice Response Task. Sustained Attention Task. *Memory tasks*- Free Recall, Delayed Recognition, Logical Reasoning Semantic Processing, Stroop Test.
Antoni et al., 1994	36, major depression/29, no major depression.		CDC criteria.	R^2 - multiple regression. Pearson r.	*Depression*- Structured Clinical Interview for DSM-III-R (SCID)Clinical Interview *Illness burden*- Sickness Impact Profile (SIP)
Johnson et al., 1994	22	21 Healthy, matched by age, education.	CDC criteria.	M ± SD.	California Verbal Learning Test (CVLT).

Table 1. (*Continued*)

Reference	N subjects	N (control)	CFS criteria	Statistical tests	Measures
Krupp et al., 1994	20	MS subjects (N unknown) healthy subjects (N unknown.)	Overwhelming fatigue for at least 6 months, with no medical origin.	M ± SD, Tukey tests, t-test.	*Depression*-The Center for Epidemiologic Studies Depression Scale. *Cognitive function*-WAIS-R: information, vocabulary. Reading-Wide Range Achievement Test Revised. *Spatial Skills*- WAIS-R: object assembly, block design. *attention*- Stoop Test, WAIS R: digit span, trail making test, digit symbol. symbol digit modalities test. *abstraction*- Booklet Category est. *Verbal memory*- Selective Reminding Test, Wechsler Memory Scale Revised, *visual memory*- Benton Visual Retention Test. *Verbal fluency*-Controlled Oral Word Association Test. *Motor speed*-Finger Oscillation.
Swanink et al., 1995	88	77 healthy subjects matched by sex, age geographical area.	Criteria specified in article.	t-test, χ^2, Mann-Whitney's U-test, ANOVA.	*Fatigue*- the Checklist Individual Strength (CIS). *Depression*- Beck Depression Inventory. *Functional Impairment*- Sickness Impact Profile (SIP).
Marshall et al., 1996	27	10 atopic, 8 healthy subjects, participating in a study of the effects of Allergy Season on mood and cognitive function.	Holmes et al., 1996 criteria for CFS.	Multiple t-tests.	Simple Choice Reaction Time. Sustained Attention- Continuous Performance Test-Identical Pairs Version. *Mood rating*- Positive and Negative Affect Schedule.

ciated with other symptoms such as sleep disturbances, then CSF might serve as a model in the newly developing field of psychoneuroimmunology. With these considerations in mind we organized the conference around a few problem areas: description and understanding of the symptoms (physiological, immunological, and behavioral) involved in CFS; the medical criterion for CSF diagnosis; the epidemiology of CSF in the general population and in the geriatric population; and possible models for explaining the CSF phenomenon.

The conference was structured to allow the speakers to address the following themes, and they have been incorporated as chapters in the pages that follow.

Fukuda supplied the necessary background to understand CFS in terms of established criteria and the epidemiological aspects of CFS. **Salit** described the importance of understanding CFS in the general population. **Natelson** summarized many studies on the behavioral and research aspects of CFS patients. **Besdine** described the importance of understanding the CFS phenomena in elderly population. **Moldofsky** reviewed the neuroimmune and the endocrine aspects of CFS, with special emphasis on sleep and sleep disturbances. **Sredni** evaluated the current literature regarding the immunological findings in CFS patients. **Behan** proposed a different and novel approach to CFS, viz. the view of CFS as a condition of altered metabolism. **Kastin** offered the view of an "outsider" and summarized the conference with an integrated presentation of the status of CFS.

The editors hope that this book will advance our understanding of the phenomena of "chronic fatigue syndrome." Enhancement of our understanding should lead to further developments, both on the theoretical level (e.g., including but not limited to a better understanding of the processes within psychoneuroimmunology, immune system function, infectious disease processes, and mechanisms of sleep disturbances), and on the practical level (to design a better rational treatment for all of those who suffer from CSF).

REFERENCES

Altay, H.T., Toner, B.B., Brooker, H., Abbey, S.E., Salit, I.E., Garfinkel, P.E. (1990) The neuropsychological dimensions of postinfectious neuromyasthenia (Chronic Fatigue Syndrome): A preliminary report. *International Journal of Psychiatry in Medicine*, 2, 141–149.

Antoni, M.H., Brickman, A., Lutgendorf, S., Kilmas, N., Imia-Fins, A., Ironson, G., Quilian, R., Miguez, M.J., Riel, F., Morgan, R., Patarca, R., Fletcher, M.A.(1994) Psychosocial correlates of illness burden in chronic fatigue syndrome. *Clinical Infectious Diseases*, 18, 73–78

Bonner, D., Ron, M., Chalder, T., Butler, S., Wessely, S. (1994) Chronic fatigue syndrome: a follow up study. *Journal of Neurology, Neurosurgery, and Psychiatry*, 57, 617–621.

Butler, S., Chalder, T., Ron, M., Wessely. (1991) Cognitive behaviour therapy in chronic fatigue syndrome. *Journal of Neurology, Neurosurgery, and Psychiatry*, 54, 153–158.

Cleare, A., Bearn, J., Allain, T., Mcgregor, A., Wessley, S., Murray, R., O'Keana, V. (1995) Contrasting neuroendocrine responses in depression and CFS. *Journal of Affective Diseases*, 35, 283–289.

Daugherty, S.A., Henry, B.E., Peterson, D.L., Swarts, R.L., Bastien, S., Thomas, R.S. (1991) Chronic fatigue syndrome in Northern Nevada. *Reviews of Infectious Diseases*,13, 39–44.

DeLuca, J., Johnson, S.K., Natelson, B.H. (1993) Information processing efficiency in chronic fatigue syndrome and multiple sclerosis. *Archives of Neurology*, 50, 301–304.

DeLuca, J., Johnson, S.K., Beldowicz, D., Natelson, B.H. (1995) Neuropsychological impairments in CFS, multiple sclerosis, and depression. *Journal of Neurology, Neurosurgery, and Psychiatry*, 58, 38–43.

Goldenberg, D.L. (1990) Fibromyalgia and chronic fatigue syndrome: Are they the same? *The Journal of Musculoskeletal Medicine*, May, 19–28.

Grafman, J., Schwartz, V., Dale, J.K., Scheffers, M., Houser, C., Straus, S.E. (1993) Analysis of neuropsychological functioning in patients with chronic fatigue syndrome. *Journal of Neurology, Neurosurgery, and Psychiatry*, 56, 684–689.

Johnson, S.K., DeLuca, J., Fiedler, N., Natelson, B.H. (1994) Cognitive functioning of patients with chronic fatigue syndrome. *Clinical Infectious Diseases*, 18, 84–85

Krupp, L.B., Sliwinski, M., Masur, D.M., Friedberg, F., Coyle, P.K. (1994) Cognitive functioning and depression in patients with chronic fatigue syndrome and multiple sclerosis. *Archives of Neurology*, 51, 705–710.

Lane, T.L., Manu, P., Mathews, D.A. (1991) Depression and somatization in the chronic fatigue syndrome. *The American Journal of Medicine*, 91, 335–343.

McDonald, E., David, A.S., Pelosi, A.J. (1993) Chronic fatigue in primary care attenders. *Psychological Medicine*, 23, 987–998.

Millenson, J. (1992) CFS: An alternative view. *Interaction*, Jan/Feb, 1–4.

Powell, R., Dolan, R., Wessley, S. (1990) Attributions and self-esteem in depression and chronic fatigue syndromes. *Journal of Psychosomatic Research*, 34, 665–673.

Ray, C., Phillips, L., Weir, W.R.C. (1993) Quality of attention in chronic fatigue syndrome: Subjective reports of everyday attention and cognitive difficulty, and performance on tasks of focused attention. (1993) *British Journal of Clinical Psychology*, 32, 357–364.

Scheffers, M.K., Johnson R., Grafman, J., Dale, J.K., Straus, S.E. (1992) Attention and short-term memory in chronic fatigue syndrome patients: an event-related potential analysis. *Neurology*, 42, 1667–1675.

Smith, A.P., Behan, P.O., Bell, W., Millar, K., Bakheit, M. (1993) Behavioural problems associated with the chronic fatigue syndrome. *British Journal of Psychology*, 84, 411–423.

Swanink, C.M.A., Vercoulen, J.H.M.M., Bleijenberg, G., Fennis, J.F., Galama, J.M.D., Van Der Meer, J.W.M. (1995) Chronic fatigue syndrome: a clinical laboratory study with a well matched control group. *Journal of Internal Medicine*, 237, 499–506.

Walford, G.A., McC Nelson, W., McCluskey, D.R. (1993) Fatigue, depression and social adjustment in chronic fatigue syndrome. *Archives of Disease in Childhood*, 68, 384–388.

While, P. (1995) The validity of fatigue syndrome that follows glandular fever. *Psychological Medicine*, 25, 917–924.

CONTENTS

1

CHRONIC FATIGUE SYNDROME IN THE ELDERLY

Another Geriatric Syndrome

Richard W. Besdine

Travelers Center on Aging
University of Connecticut Health Center School
of Medicine

Although there is a firm knowledge base emerging on chronic fatigue syndrome (CFS) in groups of patients who have been scientifically identified and carefully followed by a cadre of investigators and clinicians dedicated to the field, few have been over age 65, and fewer still among the old-old—80 years of age or older. Regrettably, it is still true that negative attitudes are common, both among the public and among health professionals, concerning aging and older adults. Although negative attitudes about aging are common, based on personal fears of the losses commonly accompanying human aging, providers of health care have additional reasons for avoiding older patients. Expectations of long and rambling complex histories, prolonged visits, multiple complaints, difficulty establishing a diagnosis, unpredictable results of treatment and complicated funding and reimbursement mechanisms for care all tend to make providers avoid older patients. Accordingly, it is

Chronic Fatigue Syndrome, edited by Yehuda and Mostofsky
Plenum Press, New York, 1997

not surprising to find that the quality of care received by older persons is less good than that received by younger adults (1).

As the science base for CSF is explored and defined, we must be meticulous as we consider applying this still-evolving disorder to older patients. Among older people, symptoms typical of CSF commonly are caused by one of the non-specific or atypical presentations of a well-defined disease entity. And whether it is malignant disease, thyroid dysfunction, hyperglycemia due to diabetes, or one of the many other disorders so common in older age, common things occur commonly in older patients and often present atypically (2,3,4).

Geriatric syndromes are the functional disabilities and non-specific presentations of disease that are so common and destructive in older persons—urinary incontinence, falls, confusional states, dizziness, unexplained weight loss, and failure to thrive (5,6). Although each has a broad differential diagnosis, comprised of many specific disorders in multiple organ systems, none in and of itself is diagnostic, nor does it dictate any specific therapy. Palliation may be possible, or even cure, but each of the syndromes demands thorough evaluation until the one cause from among many potential diseases is identified and directs treatment.

A substantial knowledge base in geriatrics and gerontology now has accumulated, allowing use of evidenced-based medicine in care of older persons with the confidence and regularity that characterizes medicine for young and middle-aged adults. Use of the knowledge base concerning clinical care of older persons in diagnosis and treatment ensures that errors of commission or omission will be minimized, to the benefit of patients. Latching on to a diagnosis of CFS in a frail older person without comprehensive assessment first represents the worst of premature closure. Valid studies have defined the changes produced by normal human aging in cardiac output, renal function, blood pressure, pulmonary capacity, sexual and immune function, skin integrity and vulnerability, glucose metabolism and virtually all other physiologic, psychologic and socioeconomic capacities in healthy older adults. When illness coincides with these and other age-related changes, the usual presentation, clinical course, response to therapy and complications and outcomes are different from those in younger persons (7). These alterations in the usual phenomenology of disease may lead clinicians to attribute puzzling symptoms to CSF rather than to seek out through comprehensive assessment the underlying causes.

It is particularly dangerous when physicians not familiar with the details of age-related change evaluate problems in an older person. Assigning abnormalities detected on physical examination or in laboratory or other diagnostic testing to normal aging when the finding is due to disease results in neglect of treatable conditions. Alternatively, if age-related changes are labeled as disease, diligent treatment attempts will almost surely end in iatrogenic harm. A third and worst outcome is the shunning of elderly patients by clinicians, frustrated and discouraged by aged patients, whose multiple problems have both disease and age-related components.

PRINCIPLES OF EVALUATION

Illness Behavior

Behavior of the Patient. Behavior of the patient is influenced by a variety of social, ethnic, psychological and clinical phenomena, including perceived severity of illness, degree of disruption of daily life alternatives to explain symptoms (denial), and the availability of care (8). Old age further alters health and illness behavior; accordingly, clinicians must understand these influences. The peer group in which the patient lives and functions and its norms and expectations concerning health has major effects. A healthy older person living in a community among similarly robust older adults is likely to evaluate as far more serious any illness, and especially a disabling one, than a nursing home resident. (9,10).

Health expectations appear to diminish as we age, independent of health status. Overestimating healthiness, called "normalization", results in attribution of dysfunction to a transient or external occurrence rather than to disease. In addition, older people tend to minimize severity of disease when finally acknowledging illness. Previous interactions with physicians in which complaints have not been taken seriously also may influence self-evaluation of health and cause delay in seeking care. The expectation of disability and functional decline in late life is likely to result in underemphasis of symptom severity and delay in treatment for improvable conditions. Attitudes of helplessness, and consequent inaction regarding health, appear to characterize current cohorts of older persons (11).

It has been widely reported that legitimate symptoms of serious but often treatable disease are concealed, or at least not reported, by elderly patients. The earliest reports came from Scotland (6), and subsequent corroborating studies from most industrialized countries documented substantial unreported illnesses and disability among elderly persons (12,13).

Although older persons have the highest baseline levels of health-promoting behavior, they appear least likely to act when experiencing symptoms of serious illness. Mild symptoms are usually attributed to age alone by individuals of all ages; but all symptoms are increasingly attributed to aging by those of increasing age. Symptoms attributed to aging usually evoked one of the following responses: 1) waiting and watching, 2) accepting the symptoms; 3) denying or minimizing the threat; or 4) postponing or avoiding medical attention (14).

Older people perceive and comprehend pain, malaise, and disability adequately, but do not report symptoms and thus do not get evaluation and treatment. A common explanation for nonreporting is the belief by older persons that old age itself brings irremediable, functional decline and feeling sick. This view makes it likely that older persons experiencing the same symptoms that bring middle-aged patients to the doctor will not seek care, will silently suffer as disease progresses, and be burdened with the functional losses of untreated illness. Sick old people are sick because they are sick, not because they are old. Although decline in some biologic functions accompanies normal human aging, these declines and their functional impact are gradual; and their impact is further softened by the decades over which they occur and by remaining, if shrinking, physiologic reserve. Major functional decline occurring abruptly in an already aged person should be assumed to be caused by disease, not aging. In addition to ageism, depression or dementia also can disrupt accurate reporting of symptoms. The increasing prevalence of cognitive loss in old age interferes with detection of disease in two ways. First, demented patients complain less specifically, and second, they also tend to let less evaluation even when they do complain.

Behavior of Disease. Multiple pathology, or the clustering of diseases and problems in one older person, is a common characteristic of illness in old age; it is highly relevant to patient evaluation and puts elderly patients at risk for functional decline due to late disease detection (15). Several or numerous concurrent problems in one older person can devastate health and functional status in several ways. First, unidentified problems are likely to influence one another and cause harm through disease-disease interactions. These interactions are especially common and dangerous in frail elderly patients, in whom major functional losses can become permanent in spite of eventual detection and treatment of the multiple problems. The late diagnosis of treatable problems whose interaction and neglect have produced permanent functional deficits is a discouraging but preventable part of geriatric care.

Second, problems which are undetected can interact with diagnostic studies or treatment of a diagnosed problem and produce iatrogenic harm through disease-treatment interactions. Careful consideration of all coexisting problems and their treatments before initiating new treatment for another is a cardinal rule of geriatric care. The number of problems per person is directly proportional to age, and rises to more than ten in the oldest and frailest, especially in the nursing home.

Functional loss is the final common pathway for many disorders in older persons. Functional impairment means decreased ability to meet one's own needs, and is measured by assessing activities of daily living (ADL), including mobility, bathing, dressing and grooming, toileting (continence) transferring, and eating (16); and by assessing instrumental activities of daily living (IADL), including housekeeping, cooking, shopping, banking, telephoning and driving or using public transportation (17). In addition, objective assessments of cognition and behavior, and of social, economic and emotional state are required to document health-related function of older persons. Unlike young persons, when elderly individuals get sick, the first sign of new illness or reactivated chronic disease is rarely a single, specific complaint which helps to localize the organ system or tissue in which the disease occurs. Instead, elderly persons usually present when ill with one or more non-specific problems, which themselves are manifestations of impaired function. These problems quickly impair independence in the previously self-sufficient elder without necessarily producing obvious, typical signs of illness by most lay and even general professional standards.

Why disease in older persons presents first with functional loss is not well understood. Disruption of homeostasis by any disease seems to be expressed most often in most vulnerable, most delicately balanced systems in previously independent, functional elderly persons. And these most vulnerable systems, or weakest links, are likely to fail and produce problems of ADL or IADL function rather than the usual classic signs and symptoms of disease. Difficulties in mobility, cognition, continence and nutrition are frequently the first manifestations of disease in an old person, regardless of the organ system or tissue in which the disease resides. Progressive restriction of the ability to maintain homeostasis, or the occurrence of "homeostenosis," is a physiological principle capsulizing much phenomenology of biological aging.

The lesson that deterioration of functional independence in active, previously unimpaired elders is an early and subtle sign of untreated illness is crucial to successful care of older persons (18,19). Disease-generated functional impairments in old people are usually treatable and improvable, but detection and evaluation are essential steps before treatment can be applied. Since disease is likely to present with abrupt impairment of function in elderly individuals, functional assessment allows early detection and thus intervention during the beginning phases of active illness (20).

PATIENT EXAMINATION

Different components of the history and physical examination need to be emphasized, and the physical environment and interpretation of laboratory data require attention as well. Perhaps most important, comprehensive functional assessment must be coupled with usual medical evaluation strategies (21,22,23).

The setting for assessment requires modification in anticipation of the common problems among older persons. Sensory impairments, physical discomfort and communication difficulties require an individualized approach to every patient regardless of age, but there are general principles useful for older patients. It is usually best to begin the interview with reassurance and introducing yourself to establish a friendly relationship; often older persons are comforted by a gentle touch on the hand or arm during conversation. The interview and examining rooms should be especially free of extraneous noise to allow communication and prevent distraction for patients with the common hearing impairment of presbycusis. Words should be spoken clearly, directly facing and level with the patient to allow lip-reading and other visual clues. Speaking louder is often helpful and necessary to communicate with a hearing-impaired older person. Since the prevalence of hearing loss exceeds 50% among patients over age 65, one should be prepared to speak up. But not all older persons are hard of hearing, and so it makes sense to ask about hearing at the outset rather than shouting unnecessarily throughout the interview (24). If hearing impairment requires raising the voice, and the deficit is due to presbycusis, which causes selective high tone loss, volume of speech should be increased in the lower frequency range rather than the high range, in which most of us tend to raise our voices. Because they are the highest pitched part of speech, presbycusis causes poor perception of consonants; in addition to speaking louder, exaggerated consonant articulation will also help. Most relevant, if the patient has a hearing aid, it should be checked for proper function be brought along to each visit.

Since visual impairment is also common among older persons, adequate lighting is important both for safety and accurate perception by the patient. It is estimated that by age 65, two-thirds of light which reaches the retina at age 20 is blocked by yellowing of the lens. Deep shadows can make a room dangerous for older individuals, but very bright light, especially from above, can be painful following cataract extraction without lens implantation. Because aging eyes accommodate less well, interviewers should never be back-lighted. As with the hearing aid, glasses should be brought to and worn at the doctor's office.

Safety and comfort require that consideration be given to equipment used in the examination. Chairs of adequate height to allow easy sitting and arising are essential. The examining table should be of a height and size so as not to endanger an unsteady, small older person in the process of mounting, dismounting or being examined. Gowns should be manageable with arthritic joints and should be short enough that an elderly woman under five feet will not step on the hem and risk a fall. Allowing sufficient time for undressing and dressing again after examination is essential, but the physician need not wait around for the patient. Since our patients are years and often decades older than their physicians and nurses, formal address as Mr., Miss, Mrs., or Ms. should be used unless the patient indicates a preference for first names. At no time should the impersonal generic "Dear" be used.

Gathering an adequate history is more complex and time-consuming in older adults, not only because they have had more time to accumulate disease, but also because disease is more common in the aged (25). In addition, more aspects of everyday life become relevant to health care in old age, and must be discussed. Besides patient interview and data from previous medical records, friends and family members, and other health professionals who have participated in care of the patient should be contacted as part of the history. Although family members can make important contributions to the history, reliance on the family or allowing them to dominate the evaluation interferes with assessment of the patient's view of the problem and of the physician's perception of cognition and emotion (26). Intellectual impairment, mild or severe, is not a reason to skip the history. Demented patients often are able to describe symptoms and response to therapy (27). The patient should be seen alone first unless there is outright refusal. Only after the patient is interviewed should the family participate.

Substantial preliminary data can be gathered before the physician sees the patient, and that information can be useful in framing additional quesstions. The "chief complaint " model usually does not work well for the complexity of disease in older patients. Often one cannot even identify a single chief complaint in an older person who is declining. Multiple problems and chronic disease generally result in numerous chronic and fluctuating unrelated complaints in the older person, usually accompanied by psychosocial disturbances. Multiple presenting complaints or identified problems are often dominated by functional losses, which are non-specific by usual disease-associated criteria. Even when a single presenting complaint can be identified in a declining older person, that complaint is less useful in narrowing the differential. Each complaint, chief or not, is likely to have its own "history of present illness" associated; and each is best enumerated separately.

Family history can usually be abbreviated in older persons, though current data on heredity of Alzheimer's disease is a notable exception. Social history must include information not usually collected in younger individuals. The social relationships with friends and family play a major role in the overall well-being and mental health of older persons, and have been shown to correlate with survival and health. Inventory of resources in the neighborhood and home, including friends, family and clergy, is needed to determine what kind and intensity of disability can be managed in the community. Services currently used and safety in the home should be documented. In view of health care costs, resources and insurance coverage should be listed. Diet history is relevant for most older individuals, especially when disease management includes food restriction or diet alteration that could interfere with nutrition; for example, diabetes, hypertension, ulcer disease or congestive heart failure. Although polio, pertussis and diphtheria immunization histories are not relevant in older persons, pneumococcal, influenza and tetanus status is important.

Sexual history is often omitted entirely by otherwise conscientious physicians, either through discomfort or mistaken assumptions about sexuality and aging. An open-ended initial question will often be sufficient (Tell me about your sex life) as long as an understanding and neutral attitude is taken in the interview (28). More specific questions about libido, masturbation, partners, frequency, function (or dysfunction), pain and satisfaction can be asked as needed. The major cause of impotence in old men is not psychological, but rather organic pathology.

Although drug lists appear regularly in an older person's medical record, believing them to be accurate and complete can be dangerous. Drugs may be duplicated when patients visit multiple physicians not known to one another, and treatment may be neglected if we assume that all listed medications are still being taken. The most reliable medication lists come from physically inspecting and inquiring about all drugs in the patient's possession. The patient and family should be asked to bring all medications to the doctor's office or to the hospital at the time of admission. With all containers laid out, both prescription and over-the-counter drugs, the physician can inquire of the patient which are taken, for what symptoms and at what intervals. Discrepancies (one kind of non-compliance) are common at any age, but occur more often and with worse consequences in older patients.

Physical Examination

Although there are a few aspects of the physical examination that require special attention in older patients, care must be taken not to make physicians feel that a great deal more must be done and time spent in examining the patient. In fact, most discourses on the special features of the physical examination in older individuals describe diseases to be found by the *usual* thorough examination which should be performed in patients of any age.

REFERENCES

1. Siu AL: The quality of medical care received by older persons. J Am Geriatric Soc 35:104, 1987.
2. Thomas FB, et al. Apathetic thyrotoxicosis: A distinctive clinical and laboratory entity. Ann Intern Med. 1970;72:679.
3. Doucet J, Trivalle Ch, Chassagne Ph, et al. Does Age Play a Role in Clinical Presentation of Hypothyroidism? J Am Geriatr Soc. 1994;42:984–986.
4. Hodkinson HM. Non-Specific presentation of illness. Br Med J. 1973;4:94.
5. Anderson WF. Personal Communication. 1972.
6. Anderson WF: The prevention of illness in the elderly: the Rutherglen experiment in medicine in old age. Proceedings of a conference held at the Royal College of Physicians of London. London: Pitman, 1966.
7. Besdine, R. W. Clinical Approach to the Elderly Patient. In Rowe, J.W., Besdine, R.W. (Eds.) *Geriatric Medicine* (2nd Ed.) 1988, Boston, MA, Little Brown and Co. 23–36.

8. Leventhal EA, Prohaska TR: Age, symptom interpretation and health behavior. J Am Geriatr Soc 34:185, 1986.
9. Levkoff SE, Cleary PD, Wetle T, Besdine RW. Illness Behavior in the Aged, Implications for Clinicians. J Am Geriatr Soc. 1988;36:622–629.
10. Levkoff SE et al: Differences in the appraisal of health between aged and middle-aged adults. J. Gerontol. 1987;42:114.
11. Besdine RW et al: Health and Illness Behaviors in Elder Veterans, in *Older Veterans: Linking VA and Community Resources*, T Wetle, JW Rowe (eds.) Cambridge: Harvard Univeristy Press, 1984.
12. Williamson J., et al. Old people at home: their unreported needs. Lancet. 1964;1:1117–1120.
13. Lyness JM, Cox C, Curry J, et.al. Older Age and the Underreporting of Depressive Symptoms. J Am Geriatr Soc. 1995;43:216–221.
14. Brody EM: Tomorrow and tomorrow and tomorrow: toward squaring the suffering curve, in *Aging 2000: Our Health Care Destiny*, Vol. II., CM Gaitz, et al (eds.), New York: Springer-Verlag, 1985.
15. Wilson LA et al: Multiple disorders in the elderly. Lancet 2:841, 1962.
16. Katz S, Ford AB, Moskowitz RW, Jackson BA, Jaffe MW. Studies of illness in the aged: the index of ADL: a standardized measure of biological and psychosocial function. JAMA 1963;185:914–9.
17. Kane, R. A., Kane, R.L. *Assessing the Elderly: A Practical Guide to Measurement*. 1981, Lexington, MA, Lexington Books.
18. American College of Physicians, Health and Public Policy Committee. Comprehensive Functional Assessment for Elderly Patients. Ann Intern Med 1988; 109:70–72.
19. National Institutes of Health Consensus Development Conference Statement: geriatric assessment methods for clinical decision-making. J Am Geriatr Soc. 1988;36:342–7.
20. Fried LP et al. Diagnosis of illness presentation in the elderly. J Am Geriatr Soc. 1991; 39:117–23.
21. Reuben DB, Siu AL. An Objective Measure of Physical Function of Elderly Outpatients, The Physical Performance Test. J Am Geriatr Soc. 1990;38:1105–1112.
22. Reuben DB, Siu AL, Kimpau S. The predictive validity of self-report and performance-based measures of function and health. J Gerontol 1992;47:M 106-M I I
23. Lachs M, Feinstein A, Cooney L, et. al. A simple procedure for general screening of functional disability in elderly patients. Ann Intern Med. 1990;112:699–706.
24. Lichtenstein MJ, Bess FH, Logan SA. Validation of Screening Tools for Identifying Hearing-Impaired Elderly in Primary Care. JAMA 1988;259:2875–2878.
25. Morley JE. Aspects of the medical history unique to older persons. JAMA 1993;269:675, 677–8.

26. Lagaay AM, van der Meij JC, Hijmans W. Validation of medical history taking as part of a population based survey in subjects aged 85 and over. BMJ. 1992;304:1091–2.
27. Davis PB, Robins, LN. History-Taking in the Elderly With and Without Cognitive Impairment. JAGS. 1989;255:37–249.
28. Bretschneider JG, McCoy NL. Sexual interest and behavior in healthy 80 to 102 year olds. Arch Sex Behav. 1988;17:109–129.

2

DEVELOPMENT OF THE 1994 CHRONIC FATIGUE SYNDROME CASE DEFINITION AND CLINICAL EVALUATION GUIDELINES

Keiji Fukuda

Influenza Branch, Division of Viral and
    Rickettsial Diseases
National Center for Infectious Diseases
Centers for Disease Control and Prevention
Atlanta, Georgia.

INTRODUCTION

A case definition is a methodologic tool that establishes criteria for classifying (in formal research) or diagnosing (in clinical practice) a case of illness or disease. Chronic fatigue syndrome (CFS) is defined solely on the basis of patient-reported symptoms and the exclusion, by clinical evaluation, of other causes of such symptoms. None of the symptoms are specific for CFS and there are no diagnostic or confirmatory laboratory tests or physical findings (Holmes, 1989; Shafran, 1991; Klonoff, 1992). Because of these limitations, published reference CFS case definitions have been crucial for coordinating research on this condition and for facilitating effective communications among investigators, physicians, and patients.

Chronic Fatigue Syndrome, edited by Yehuda and Mostofsky
Plenum Press, New York, 1997

Between 1988 and 1990, three separate CFS research case definitions were published by North American (Holmes et al., 1988), Australian (Lloyd et al., 1988; Lloyd et al., 1990), and British (Sharpe et al.,1991) groups. In 1994, a fourth CFS case definition and a set of clinical evaluation guidelines were published by an international group of researchers, which included the primary authors of the earlier publications (Fukuda et al., 1994). The major reasons for this effort were to 1) address some of the limitations of the 1988 CFS working case definition, 2) increase the coordination of CFS research among international investigators, and 3) improve the clinical evaluation of persons with unexplained severe fatigue.

BRIEF OVERVIEW OF PRECEDING EVENTS AND CONSIDERATIONS

In the early and mid-1980s, a group of studies (Tobi et al., 1982; Jones et al., 1985; Straus et al., 1985) spurred interest in the possibility of a new and distinct chronic fatiguing illness. Because these early reports suggested an association (which is no longer generally accepted) with Epstein-Barr virus (EBV) infection, names such as chronic EBV syndrome and chronic mononucleosis were coined and became popular. In 1985, a workshop at the National Institutes of Health (NIH) recognized the need for a reference case definition to coordinate a growing number of loosely related studies (Schluederberg et al., 1992). Subsequently, the Centers for Disease Control (CDC) convened a group of federal and nonfederal researchers and clinicans. In 1988, this group published a "working" CFS case definition and also unanimously recommended adoption of the name "chronic fatigue syndrome," to avoid premature implications regarding the condition's underlying cause (Holmes et al., 1988a).

The publication of the 1988 CFS working case definition was a pivotal event. It focused scientific and general attention on this condition and quickly became the standard North American CFS case definition for clinical practice and investigations. The publication of Australian (Lloyd et al., 1988; Lloyd et al., 1990) and British (Sharpe et al.,1991) CFS case definitions soon followed. Although the North American, Australian, and British approaches differed in certain respects, they represented a major advancement in the scientific standards of studies of CFS.

By 1992, however, the adequacy of the 1988 working CFS case definition was openly in question. In a succinct editorial, Straus pointed out that several issues pertaining to how CFS was defined were unresolved (Straus, 1992). These issues included 1) the lack of objective or pathognomonic criteria for CFS, 2) the vagueness of some of the criteria in the 1988 CFS working case definition, which inevitably led to differences in the interpretation and implementation of the criteria, and 3) the practical difficulty of excluding "all" other causes of protracted fatigue. Straus also pointed out that the relationship between psychiatric conditions and CFS remained uncertain and controversial (Matthews et al., 1988; Holmes et al, 1988b).

CDC CONCERNS

At the same time, related concerns were under discussion among CDC investigators. The most pressing was the fact that CFS studies had yet to show any consistent and convincing pathophysiologic findings. Moreover, studies concentrating on specific areas of potential pathology were often extremely conflicting. For example, one review of infectious and immunologic abnormalities among CFS subjects showed that many of such reported findings were highly variable at best, and extremely difficult to interpret as a group (Mawle et al., 1994). CDC investigators were concerned that one major reason for the inconsistent findings was ongoing differences in how individual investigators were selecting or defining CFS cases. Although CFS studies after 1988 frequently made mention of the 1988 CFS working case definition, informal discussions with other investigators, as well as published observations, led CDC investigators to conclude that the goal of standardized CFS cases among formal studies had not been achieved. For example, five of six researchers at a 1991 NIH workshop on CFS indicated that each modified the 1988 CFS working case definition differently (Schluederberg et al., 1992).

The ambiguity of some of the criteria in the 1988 CFS working case definition was one reason why that case definition was interpreted differently by investigators. CDC investigators also found some of the criteria difficult to implement in a consistent manner. From 1989 through 1993, CDC conducted surveillance for CFS in four U.S. cities (Reno, Nevada; Wichita, Kansas; Grand Rapids, Michigan; and Atlanta, Georgia) and used an elaborate and time-consuming process, which required the input of several physicians, to classify CFS cases (Gunn et al., 1993). Although this process represented a substantial effort to classify CFS cases as systematically and objectively as possible, it was often impossible to determine whether certain critieria in the 1988 CFS working case definition had been met. For example, deciding whether a subject's activity level had been reduced by 50% or more often required a great deal of subjective judgement.

A second concern of CDC investigators was the finding that application of the 1988 CFS working case definition did not identify a homogeneous or distinct group of cases. In the 1989–1993 CFS surveillance system, subjects classified with CFS were not clinically or demographically distinguishable from subjects whose chronic (≥6 months) fatigue did not meet CFS-defining criteria (Reyes et al, 1996). This was an important observation. The 1988 CFS working case definition had deliberately been made highly restrictive as a strategy for identifying a homogeneous and distinct group of subjects. The basic idea had been to use very restrictive criteria to define a pure group of CFS cases as a means for identifying the underlying pathophysiology. The failure to define a unique group made arguements for a less restrictive case definition more compelling. If the case definition was made less restrictive by dropping or simplifying some of the criteria, it would allow researchers to apply the CFS case definition more consistently.

A final consideration that helped to tip the decision in favor of developing the 1994 CFS case definition, was the desirability of establishing closer links among international CFS researchers. CDC investigators felt that a joint international effort to develop a single reference standard would provide a substantial step in that direction.

THE PROCESS OF DEVELOPING THE 1994 CFS CASE DEFINITION AND GUIDELINES

Between 1992 and 1994, a series of formal and informal meetings was held at CDC and NIH, which involved a group of scientists and clinicians (Appendix 1) called the "International Chronic Fatigue Syndrome Study Group" (and referred to as the "study group" in this chapter). Overall, more than 50 investigators, clinicians, and patient advocates were involved in this process. The meetings were used to identify areas of concern, to develop goals, to review published and unpublished data, and to reach a consensus on issues.

One particularly useful outcome of this process, which was unforseen at the outset, was the decision to include a set of clinical evaluation guidelines in the publication. The guidelines provide practical information on the evaluation of fatigued individuals, and stress the need to thoroughly evaluate subjects before diagnosing or classifying CFS. As presented in the publication, the CFS case definition forms one part of the total guidelines. The 1994 CFS case definition does not stand alone as an isolated set of criteria.

The impetus for developing the guidelines came from the clinicians in the study group, who universally observed that many patients with unexplained fatiguing illness were receiving either unecessary and wasteful tests, or alternatively, inadequate clinical evaluation. The latter point was underscored by a finding from the 1989–1993 CFS surveillance system (Reyes et al., 1996). Subjects could not enroll in that surveillance system unless a referring physician was unable to find the cause for the person's chronic fatigue or unwellness. Despite this requirement, the surveillance evaluation procedures showed that 18% of the 565 participants had a diagnosable disorder, at the time of entry, which potentially explained the symptoms and excluded the subject from classification as a CFS case. The procedures that were used to identify those disorders were straight forward and consisted of running a battery of routine laboratory screening tests and a review of medical records.

AN OVERVIEW OF THE GUIDELINES AND CASE DEFINITION

The evaluation guidelines, including the CFS case definition, are straightforward in concept and indicate that severe fatigue deserves a thorough clinical evaluation (which may require multiple visits). One of three general outcomes to this process is possible. First, a primary underlying disorder may be identified that categorically excludes the diagnosis of CFS. Second, a number of conditions may be identified that do not preclude the diagnosis of CFS. Third, no diagnosable condition may be found, in which case the classification or diagnosis of CFS may be appropriate if all of the inclusion critiera have been met.

At this point, the guidelines distinguish between the concerns of clinicans, who are primarily focused on the care of patients, and investigators working in the setting of a formal study. In the setting of a formal study, subjects with unexplained chronic fatigue that does not meet CFS criteria can grouped in a category termed "idiopathic chronic fatigue." The sole purpose of this category, which does not establish a new clinical entity, is to encourage researchers to clarify the key issue of whether CFS is substantially different from less-defined chronic fatigue. This is an important issue for understanding CFS. Finally, the guidelines encourage researchers to divide CFS and idiopathic chronic fatigue subjects into subgroups for comparison.

COMMENTARY ON INDIVIDUAL SECTIONS OF THE GUIDELINES

The Clinical Evaluation

Until a diagnostic marker is available, the diagnosis of CFS will remain one of exclusion. The purpose of the clinical evaluation is to identify any factors contributing to the person's symptoms, and particularly, any disorders that exclude the diagnosis of CFS.. During the interview, particular attention should be paid to events at the onset of the fatigue and current level of activities. In addition, the interview should explcitly cover the use of medications, alcohol and other potentially addictive substances, as well as unusual dietary supplements.

The need to search for psychologic abnormalities, which may constitute the primary reason for the subject's symptoms, or act as contributing factors, cannot be overstressed. The most important of these conditions is major depression, which is significantly more prevalent in populations defined by fatigue (Manu et al., 1988) and CFS (Kruesi et al., 1989; Wessely & Powell, 1989)) than in the general population. While a majority of the working group felt that a formal psychiatric evaluation by a specialist was desirable, general implementation of such a recommendation was thought to be impractical. Therefore, the guidelines recommend a mental status examination, which can be performed by any general health care practitioner, as a minimum acceptable level of evaluation.

The purpose of the physical examination and screening laboratory tests is to identify any finding that may point to another diagnosable disorder as the cause for the subject's symptoms. The guidelines stress, in no uncertain terms, the lack of physical or laboratory findings for confirming or diagnosisng CFS. In practice, most routine physical and laboratory test examinations among such persons yield normal results or minor abnormalities (Kroenke et al., 1988; Lane et al., 1990)

Conditions That Exclude Chronic Fatigue Syndrome

The clinical evaluation process may identify several diagnosable disorders, some of which should be considered the primary cause for the person's symptoms and preclude further consideration of CFS. Because an exhaustive listing of all such disorders was considered impractical, five general categories were presented in the guidelines instead.

The first group of disorders that excludes the diagnosis of CFS is active major medical conditions, which are normally associated with fatigue (Kroenke, 1989). This group of diseases is self-explanatory. The second category of disorders is less categorical and more complicated. A number of major medical conditions have the capacity for resolving permanently or becoming active after variable periods of quiesence. Examples include hepatitis B virus infection and certain malignancies. If such a condition has been documented in the past, then the permanent resolution or cure of the condition should be adequately established, according to accepted clinical standards, before the diagnosis or classification of CFS can be made. For example, hepatitis B virus infection may resolve permanently or lead to chronic disease. If hepatitis B virus infection was diagnosed in the past, then the presence of hepatitis B surface antibody should be documented as proof that the infection has resolved. A more vexing situtation is posed by some major malignancies. In some instances, the treatment of a major malignancy may be considered curative, depending on the tumor stage at treatment. In such a situation, the diagnosis of CFS may be appropriate. However, in the many instances where the longterm outcome is uncertain, even after a substantial disease-free period, the diagnosis of CFS is unacceptable.

A group of severe psychiatric and neurologic conditions (i.e., major depressive disorder with psychotic or melancholic features, bipolar affective disorders, schizophrenia of any subtype, delusional disorders of any subtype, dementias of any subtype, anorexia nervosa, and bulimia nervosa) comprises the third category. These particular disorders were singled out for several reasons. First, each is a severe and chronic illness that makes the assessment of "unexplained" symptoms extremely difficult. Even more importantly, the study group noted that specific therapies were available for these conditions and felt that the risk of diverting attention away from their treatment, by making a diagnosis of CFS, was unacceptable. Finally, each of these disorders is not generally known to be associated with CFS.

The fourth category consists of substance abuse, which is self-explanatory. The fifth category is comprised of severe obesity, another condition that highlights the difficulty of assessing the presence of "unexplained" symptoms, such as fatigue or joint pains, in certain situtations. This section of the guidelines concludes by pointing out that test abnormalities strongly suggestive of an exclusionary condition should be resolved before making a diagnosis of CFS.

Conditions That Are Compatible with Chronic Fatigue Syndrome

In contrast to the types of disorders just discussed, many conditions do not preclude the diagnosis of CFS and can be considered comorbid conditions. The guidelines also group these conditions into one of several categories. The first and most important group of such disorders is other symptom-defined illnesses that cannot be confirmed by laboratory tests. This category includes psychiatric conditions (other than the ones that categorically exclude CFS) of which the most important is major depression (without psychosis or melancholia). Other examples include fibromyalgia (Goldenberg, 1987).

There were three main reasons why the study group decided that the presence of other symptom-based diagnoses did not preclude the diagnosis or classification of CFS. First, CFS shows considerable overlap with several symptom-defined disorders, such as major depression (Kruesi et al., 1989; Wessely & Powell, 1989) and fibromyalgia (Buchwald et al., 1987). Subjects who meet criteria for CFS also often meet diagnostic criteria for major depression or fibromyalgia. However, the relationship between CFS and these other disorders is unclear. On the one hand, it is possible that CFS, fibromyalgia, and major depression are distinct entities that happen to overlap with each other. However, it is also possible that many of the distinctions made among such disorders largely are artifactual and primarily reflect the biases of different medical disciplines. Until this issue is settle, the study group saw no *a priori* reason for why the diagnosis of CFS was incompatible with another symptom-defined disorder. Finally, the exclusion of subjects with certain of these diagnoses, particularly major depression, was felt to be practically impossible. The removal of major depression as an exclusionary condition marked a distinct change from the 1988 CFS working case definition but was consistent with recommendations from the 1991 NIH CFS work shop (Schluederberg at al., 1992).

Classification of Cases

A subject whose fatiguing illness has persisted for at least six months and remained unexplained after appropriate evlauation is eligible for further classification as either a case of CFS or idiopathic chronic fatigue.

CHRONIC FATIGUE SYNDROME

The 1994 revised CFS case definition was modeled on the 1988 CFS working case definition. Some features of the 1988 CFS working case definition were retained or dropped with little dissent in the study group. For example, the requirement for at least 6 months of fatigue was retained to facilitate comparison with earlier CFS cases. All physical signs were dropped as inclusion criteria because the verification of those criteria was universally regarded as unreliable. The requirement for an "average daily activity below 50%" also was eliminated because verification of this level of impairment was felt to be difficult and unreliable.

A great deal of discussion focused on ways to improve the operational definition of fatigue, a problem that has long plagued other investigators (Barofsky & Legro, 1991; Lewis & Wessely, 1992). The study group grappled with two major issues. The first was how to convey the sense of fatigue felt to be characterisitc of CFS. In the 1994 CFS case definition article, the fatigue of CFS was described as "severe mental and physical exhaustion, which differs from somnolence or lack of motivation, and which is not attributable to exertion or another diagnosable disease." Most of the study group agreed with this concept. The second issue was how to capture the sense of a symptom's severity, specifically in relation to fatigue but also the neurocognitive symptoms (i.e., impairment in short-term memory or concentration). Although several approaches were discussed, including the use of scales and other instruments, the study group opted to operationalize severity by requiring a diminishment in previous levels of "occupational, educational, social, or personal" activity.

The one issue that generated the most discussion and disagreement among the working group was whether to retain symptom criteria other than chronic fatigue. Some members favored retaining all or most of the symptom criteria in the 1988 CFS working case definition because it was felt that retention of such symptoms reflected the distinctive sense of CFS. However, no data were available that convincingly suggested that any symptom criteria made the definition of CFS more precise or valid.

By contrast, other members favored the deletion of all of the symptom criteria, other than fatigue. There were two main lines of argument. First, it was argued that no study had shown that any of the symptoms, alone or in combination, were specific for CFS. Second, some studies had suggested that a requirement for multiple symptoms in the CFS case definition biased it toward the selection of persons with psychiatric disorders (Katon & Russo, 1992). At the end of these discussions, a pragmatic compromise was reached in which the list of symptom criteria was decreased from 11 to eight and the required number of symptoms was decreased from eight to four.

IDIOPATHIC CHRONIC FATIGUE

This category consists of persons whose chronic fatigue is not explained by any diagnosable disorders but also does not meet CFS-defining criteria. The status of this group of subjects is unknown. The purpose of categorizing them is to emphasize the need to determine the relation between this type of fatigue and CFS.

SUBGROUPING OF CASES IN FORMAL STUDIES

The study group recommended the subgrouping of cases (CFS and idiopathic fatigue) in formal studies as a means for searching for important subpopulations of fatigue cases. For example, the guidelines suggest that one way to subgroup CFS cases is by the presence or absence of major depression. This is a practical approach for determining whether CFS cases with major depression differ from CFS cases without major depression. Moreover, it is an approach for controlling for the effects of potential confounding. For example, in studies of immunologic abnormalities among CFS cases, dividing CFS cases on the basis of the presence or absence of major depression will help to resolve whether major depression is a confounding factor

associated with any possible abnormal immunologic results.

SUMMARY

The definition of CFS can be expected to remain in a
state of flux until an objective test is developed. The criteria
will undoubtedly change through an iterative process as
more information on the condition becomes available. Given
these realities, the 1994 guidelines and CFS case definition
represent a scientifically valid and comprehensive approach
toward addressing many of the issues presented by attempts
to define an entity such as CFS. The discussion in this article should make it clear that the decisions made by the
study group were usually guided by practical concerns as
well as the underlying desire to improve the quality of research on CFS and related conditions.

The guidelines and case definition do not constitute a
"defnitive" statement; however, it is hoped that they provide CFS patients, health care workers, and researchers
with a common point of reference that will facilitate better
and more direct communications with each other.

APPENDIX 1. INTERNATIONAL CHRONIC FATIGUE SYNDROME STUDY GROUP MEMBERS

Keiji Fukuda	Simon Wessely	Jan H.M.M. Vercoulen
Stephen E. Straus	Nelson M. Gantz	Umberto Tirelli
Ian Hickie	Gary P. Holmes	Birgitta Evengard
Michael C. Sharpe	Dedra Buchwald	Benjamin H. Natelson
James G. Dobbins	Susan Abbey	Lea Steele
Anthony Komaroff	Jonathan Rest	Michele Reyes
Ann Schluederberg	Jay A. Levy	William C. Reeves
James F. Jones	Heidi Jolsn	
Andrew R. Lloyd	Daniel L. Peterson	

APPENDIX 2. GUIDELINES FOR THE CLINICAL EVALUATION AND STUDY OF THE CHRONIC FATIGUE SYNDROME AND OTHER ILLNESSES ASSOCIATED WITH UNEXPLAINED CHRONIC FATIGUE (ADAPTED FROM *ANNALS OF INTERNAL MEDICINE*, 1994;121:953–959)

Definition and Clinical Evaluation of Prolonged Fatigue and Chronic Fatigue

Prolonged fatigue is defined as self-reported, persistent fatigue lasting 1 month or longer. Chronic fatigue is defined as self-reported persistent or relapsing fatigue lasting 6 or more consecutive months.

The presence of prolonged or chronic fatigue requires clinical evaluation to identify underlying or contributing conditions that require treatment. Further diagnosis or classification of chronic fatigue cases cannot be made without such an evaluation. The following items should be included in the clinical evaluation.

1. A thorough history that covers medical and psychosocial circumstances at the onset of fatigue; depression or other psychiatric disorders; episodes of medically unexplained symptoms; alcohol or other substance abuse; and current use of prescription and over-the-counter medications and food supplements.

2. A mental status examination to identify abnormalities in mood, intellectual function, memory, and personality. Particular attention should be directed toward current symptoms of depression or anxiety, self-destructive thoughts, and observable signs such as psychomotor retardation. Evidence of a psychiatric or neurologic disorder requires that an appropriate psychiatric, psychological, or neurologic evaluation be done.

3. A thorough physical examination.

4. A minimum battery of laboratory screening tests
   including complete blood count with leukocyte differential; erythrocyte sedimentation rate; serum
   levels of alanine aminotransferase, total protein, albumin, globulin, alkaline phosphatase, calcium,
   phosphorus, glucose, blood urea nitrogen, electrolytes, and creatinine; determination of thyroid-
   stimulating hormone; and urinalysis.

Routinely doing other screening tests for all patients
has no known value. However, further tests may be indicated on an individual basis to confirm or exclude another
diagnosis. such as multiple sclerosis. In these cases, additional tests or procedures should be done according to accepted clinical standards.

The use of tests to diagnose the chronic fatigue syndrome (rather than to exclude other diagnostic possibilities) should be done only in the setting of protocol-based
research. The fact that such tests are investigational and
do not aid in diagnosis or management should be explained to the patient.

In clinical practice, no additional tests, including laboratory tests and neuroimaging studies, can be recommended for the specific purpose of diagnosing the chronic
fatigue syndrome. Tests should be directed toward confirming or excluding other etiologic possibilities. Examples
of specific tests that do not confirm or exclude the diagnosis of the chronic fatigue syndrome include serologic
tests for Epstein-Barr virus, retroviruses, human herpesvirus 6, enteroviruses, and *Candida albicans;* tests of immunologic function, including cell population and function
studies; and imaging studies, including magnetic resonance imaging scans and radionuclide scans (such as sin-
gle-photon emission computed tomography and positron
emission tomography) of the head.

Conditions That Explain Chronic Fatigue

The following conditions exclude a patient from the diagnosis of unexplained chronic fatigue.

1. Any active medical condition that may explain the presence of chronic fatigue (Kroenke, 1989), such as untreated hypothyroidism, sleep apnea, and narcolepsy, and iatrogenic conditions such as side effects of medication.

2. Any previously diagnosed medical condition whose resolution has not been documented beyond reasonable clinical doubt and whose continued activity may explain the chronic fatiguing illness. Such conditions may include previously treated malignancies and unresolved cases of hepatitis B or C virus infection.

3. Any past or current diagnosis of a major depressive disorder with psychotic or melancholic features; bipolar affective disorders; schizophrenia of any subtype; delusional disorders of any subtype; dementias of any subtype; anorexia nervosa; or bulimia nervosa.

4. Alcohol or other substance abuse within 2 years before the onset of the chronic fatigue and at any time afterward.

5. Severe obesity (Kuczmarski, 1992; Bray, 1992) as defined by a body mass index [body mass index= weight in kilograms/(height in meters)2] equal to or greater than 45.

Any unexplained physical examination finding or laboratory or imaging test abnormality that strongly suggests the presence of an exclusionary condition must be resolved before further classification.

Conditions That Do Not Adequately Explain Chronic Fatigue

The following conditions do not exclude a patient from the diagnosis of unexplained chronic fatigue.

1. Any condition defined primarily by symptoms that cannot be confirmed by diagnostic laboratory tests, including fibromyalgia, anxiety disorders, somato-

form disorders, nonpsychotic or nonmelancholic depression, neurasthenia, and multiple chemical sensitivity disorder.

2. Any condition under specific treatment sufficient to alleviate all symptoms related to that condition and for which the adequacy of treatment has been documented. Such conditions include hypothyroidism for which the adequacy of replacement hormone has been verified by normal thyroid-stimulating hormone levels or asthma in which the adequacy of treatment has been determined by pulmonary function and other testing.

3. Any condition, such as Lyme disease or syphilis, that was treated with definitive therapy before development of chronic symptomatic sequelae.

4. Any isolated and unexplained physical examination finding or laboratory or imaging test abnormality that is insufficient to strongly suggest the existence of an exclusionary condition. Such conditions include an elevated antinuclear antibody titer that is inadequate to strongly support a diagnosis of a discrete connective tissue disorder without other laboratory or clinical evidence.

Major Classification Categories: Chronic Fatigue Syndrome and Idiopathic Chronic Fatigue

Clinically evaluated, unexplained cases of chronic fatigue can be separated into either the chronic fatigue syndrome or idiopathic chronic fatigue on the basis of the following criteria.

A case of the chronic fatigue syndrome is defined by the presence of the following: 1) clinically evaluated, unexplained, persistent or relapsing chronic fatigue that is of new or definite onset (has not been lifelong); is not the result of ongoing exertion; is not substantially alleviated by rest; and results in substantial reduction in previous levels of occupational, educational, social, or personal activities; and 2) the concurrent occurrence of four or more of the following symptoms, all of which must have persisted or recurred during 6 or more consecutive months of illness and must not have predated the fatigue: self-reported impairment in short-term memory or concentration severe enough to cause substantial reduction in previous levels of occupational, educational, social, or personal activities; sore throat; tender cervical or axillary lymph nodes; muscle pain, multijoint pain without joint swelling or redness; headaches of a new type, pattern, or severity; unrefreshing sleep; and postexertional malaise lasting more than 24 hours.

The method used (for example, a predetermined checklist developed by the investigator or spontaneous reporting by the study participant) to establish the presence of these and any other symptoms should be specified.

A case of idiopathic chronic fatigue is defined as clinically evaluated, unexplained chronic fatigue that fails to meet criteria for the chronic fatigue syndrome. The reasons for failing to meet the criteria should be specified.

Subgrouping and Stratification of Major Classification Categories

In formal studies, cases of the chronic fatigue syndrome and idiopathic chronic fatigue should be subgrouped before analysis or stratified during analysis by the presence or absence of essential variables, which should be routinely established in all studies. Further subgrouping by optional variables can be done according to specific reearch interests.

Essential Subgrouping Variables

1. Any clinically important coexisting medical or neuropsychiatric condition that does not explain the chronic fatigue. The presence or absence, classification, and timing of onset of neuropsychiatric conditions should be established using published or freely available instruments, such as the Com-

posite International Diagnostic Instrument (Robins et al., 1988), the National Institute of Mental Health Diagnostic Interview Schedule (Robins et al., 1981), and the Structured Clinical Interview for DSM-III(R) (Spitzer et al., 1992).

2. Current level of fatigue, including subjective or performance aspects. These levels should be measured using published or widely available instruments. Examples include instruments by Schwartz and colleagues (Schwartz et al., 1993), Piper and colleagues (Piper et al., 1989), Krupp and colleagues (Krupp et al., 1989), Chalder and colleagues (Chalder et al., 1993), and Vercoulen and colleagues (Vercoulen et al., 1994).

3. Total duration of fatigue.

4. Current level of overall functional performance as measured by published or widely available instruments, such as the Medical Outcomes Study Short Form 36 (Ware & Sherbourne, 1992) and the Sickness Impact Profile (Bergner et al., 1981).

Optional Subgrouping Variables

Examples of optional variables include:

1. Epidemiologic or laboratory features of specific interest to researchers. Examples include laboratory documentation or self-reported history of an infectious illness at the onset of fatiguing illness, a history of rapid onset of illness, or the presence or level of a particular immunologic marker.

2. Measurements of physical function quantified by means such as treadmill testing or motion-sensing devices.

REFERENCES

Barofsky, I. & Legro, M.W. (1991). Definition and measurement of fatigue. Rev Infect Dis, 13(Suppl l), S94-S97.

Bergner, M., Bobbin, R.A., Carter, W.B. & Gilson, B.S. (1981). The Sickness Impact Profile: development and final revision of a health status measure. Med Care, XIX, 787–805.

Bray, G.A. (1992). Pathophysiology of obesity. Am J Clin Nutr, 55(2 Suppl), 488S-494S.

Buchwald, D., Goldenberg, D.L., Sullivan, J.L. & Komaroff, A.L. The "chronic, active Epstein-Barr virus infection" syndrome and primary fibromyalgia. Arthritis Rheum, 30, 1132–1136.

Chalder, T., Berelowitz, G., Pawlikowska, T., Watts, L., Wessely, S. & Wright, D. & Wallace, E.P. (1993). Development of a fatigue scale. Psychosom Res, 37, 147–153.

Fukuda, K., Straus, S.E., Hickie, I., Sharpe, M.C., Dobbins, J.G., Komaroff, A. & the International Chronic Fatigue Syndrome Group (1994). The chronic fatigue syndrome: a comprehensive approach to its definition and study. Ann Intern Med, 121, 953–959.

Goldenberg, D.L. (1987). Firbromyalgia syndrome. An emerging but controversial condition. J Am Med Assoc, 257, 2782–2787.

Gunn, W.J., Connell, D.B. & Randall, B. (1993). Epidemiology of chronic fatigue syndrome: the Centers for Disease Control study. In: G. Bock & J. Whelan (Eds.), Chronic Fatigue Syndrome. (pp. 83–101). New York: Wiley.(Ciba Foundation Symposium 173).

Holmes, G.P., Kaplan, J.E., Gantz, N.M., Komaroff, A.L., Schonberger, L.B., Straus, S.E., Jones, J.F., Dubois, R.E., Cunningham-Rundles, C., Pahwa, S., Tosato, G., Zegans, L.S., Purtilo, D.T., Brown, N., Schooley, R.T. & Brus, I. (1988a). Chronic fatigue syndrome: a working case definition. Ann Intern Med, 108, 387–389.

Holmes, G.P., Kaplan, J.E., Schonberger, L.B., Straus, S.E., Zegans, L.S., Gantz, N.M., Brus, I., Komaroff, A., Jones, J.F., Dubois, R.E., Cunningham-Rundles, C., Tosato, G., Brown, N.A., Pahwa, S. & Schooley, R.T. (1988b). Definition of the chronic fatigue syndrome [Letter]. Ann Intern Med, 109, 512.

Holmes, G.P. (1989). The chronic fatigue syndrome. In: D. Schlossberg (Ed.), Infectious Mononucleosis. 2nd ed. (Pp. 172–193). New York: Springer-Verlag.

Jones, J.F., Ray, C.G., Minnich, L.L., Hicks, M.J., Kibler, R. & Lucas, D.O. (1985). Evidence for active Epstein-Barr virus infection in patients with persistent, unexplained illness: elevated anti-early antigen antibodies. Ann Intern Med, 102, 1–7.

Katon, W. & Russo, J. (1992). Chronic fatigue syndrome criteria. A critique of the requirement for multiple physical complaints. Arch Intem Med, 152, 1604–1609.

Klonoff, D.C. (1992). Chronic fatigue syndrome. Clin Infect Dis, 15, 812–823.

Kroenke, K., Wood, D.R., Mangelsdorf, A.D., Meier, N.J. & Powell, J.B. (1988). Chronic fatigue in primary care. Prevalence, patient characteristics, and outcome. J Amer Med Assoc, 206, 929–934.

Kroenke, K. (1989). Chronic fatigue: frequency, causes, evaluation, and managenent. Compr Ther, 15, 3–7.

Kruesi, M.J., Dale, J. & Straus, S.E. (1989). Psychiatric diagnoses in patients who have chronic fatigue syndrome. J Clin Psychiatry, 50, 53–56.

Krupp, L.B., LaRocca, N.G., Muir-Nash, J. & Steinberg, A.D. (1989). The fatigue severity scale. Application to patients with multiple sclerosis and systemic lupus erythematosus. Arch Neurol, 46, 1121–1123.

Kuczmarski, R.J. (1992). Prevalence of overweight and weight gain in the United States. Am J Clin Nutr, 55(2 Suppl), 495S-502S.

Lane, T.J., Matthews, D.A. & Manu, P. (1990). The low yield of physical examinations and laboratory investigations of patients with chronic fatigue. Am J Med Sci, 299, 313–318.

Lewis, G. & Wessely, S. (1992). The epidemiology of fatigue: more questions than answers. J Epidemiol Community Health, 46, 92–97.

Lloyd, A.R., Wakefield, D., Boughton, C. & Dwyer J. (1988). What is myalgic encephalomyelitis? [Letter]. Lancet, 1, 1286–1287.

Lloyd, A.R., Hickie, I., Boughton, C.R., Spencer, O. & Wakefield, D. (1990). Prevalence of chronic fatigue syndrome in an Australian population. Med J Aust, 153, 522–528.

Manu, P., Matthews, D.A. & Lane, T.J. (1988). The mental health of patients with a chief complaint of chronic fatigue. A prospective evaluation and follow-up. Arch Intern Med, 148, 2213–2217.

Matthews, D.A., Lane, T.J. & Manu, P. (1988). Definition of the chronic fatigue syndrome [Letter]. Ann Intern Med, 109, 511–512.

Mawle, A.C., Reyes, M. & Schmid, D.S. (1994). Is chronic fatigue syndrome an infectious disease? Infect Agents Dis, 2, 333–341.

Piper, B.F., Lindsey, A.M., Dodd, M.J., Perketich, S., Paul, S.M. & Weller, S. The development of an instrument to measure the subjective dimension of fatigue. (1989). In: S.G. Funk, P.M. Tournquist, M.T. Campagne, L. Archer Gopp, R.A. Wiese, (Eds), *Key Aspects of Comfort. Management of Pain, Fatigue and Nausea* (pp. 199–208). New York: Springer.

Reyes, M., Gary, H.E., Dobbins, J.G., Randall, B., Steele, L., Fukuda, K., Holmes, G.P., Connell, D.G., Mawle, A.C., Schmid, D.S., Stewart, J.A., Schonberger, L.B., Gunn, W.J. & Reeves, W.C. (1996). Descriptive epidemiology of chronic fatigue syndrome: CDC surveillance in four U.S. cities. Morbid Mortal Wkly Rep CDC. Surveillance Summaries, (In-press).

Robins, L.N., Heizer, J.E., Croughan, J. & Ratcliff, K.S. (1981). National Institute of Mental Health Diagnostic Inteniew Schedule. Its history, characteristics, and validity. Arch Gen Psychiatry, 38, 381–389.

Robins LN, Wine J. Wittchen HU, Heizer JE, Babor TF, Burke J, Farmer A, Jablenski A, Pickens, R, Regier, D.A., Sartorius, N. & Towle,

L.H. (1988). The Composite International Diagnostic Inteniew. An epidemiologic instrument suitable for use in conjunction with different diagnostic systems and in different cultures. Arch Gen Psychiatry, 45, 1069–1077.

Schwartz, J.E., Jandorf, L. & Krupp, L.B. (1993). The measurement of fatigue: a new instrument. J Psychosom Res, 37, 753–762.

Schluederberg, A., Straus, S.E., Peterson, P., Blumenthal, S., Komaroff, A.L., Spring, S.B., Landay, L. & Buchwald, D. (1992). NIH conference. Chronic fatigue syndrome research. Definition and medical outcome assessment. Ann Intern Med, 117, 325–331.

Shafran, S.D. (1991). The chronic fatigue syndrome. Am J Med, 90, 730–739.

Sharpe, M.C., Archard, L.C., Banatvala, J.E., Borysiewicz, L.K., Clare, A.W., David, A., Edwards, R.H.T., Hawton, K.E.H., Lambert, H.P., Lane, R.J.M., McDonald, E.M., Mowbray, J.F., Pearson, D.J., Peto, T.E.A., Preedy, V.R., Smith, A.P., Smith, D.G., Taylor, D.J., Tyrell, D.A.J., Wessely, S., White, P.D., Behan, P.O., Clifford Rose, F., Peters, T.J., Wallace, P.G., Warrell, D.A. & Wright, D.J.M. (1991). A report--chronic fatigue syndrome: guidelines for research. J R Soc Med, 84, 118–121.

Spitzer, R.L., Williams, J.B., Gibbon, M. & First, M.B. (1992). The Structured Clinical Interiew for DSM-HI-R (SCID). 1: History, rationale, and description. Arch Gen Psychiatr, 49, 624–629.

Straus, S.E., Tosato, G., Armstrong, G., Lawley, T., Preble, O.T., Henle, W., Davey, R., Pearson, G., Epstein, J., Brus, I. & Blaese R.M. (1985). Persisting illness and fatigue in adults with evidence of Epstein-Barr virus infection. Ann Intern Med, 102, 7–16.

Straus, S.E. (1992). Defining the chronic fatigue syndrome [Editorial]. Arch Intern Med, 152, 1569–1570.

Tobi, M., Morag, A., Ravid, Z., Chowers, I., Feldman-Weiss, V., Michaeli, Y., Ben-Chetrit, E. & Shalit, M. (1982). Prolonged atypical illness associated with serological evidence of persistent Epstein-Barr virus infection. Lancet, 1, 61–64.

Vercoulen, J.H., Swanink, C.M., Fennis, J.F., Galama, J.M., Van der Meer, J.W. & Bleijenberg, G. (1994). Dimensional assessment of chronic fatigue syndrome. J Psychosom Res, 38, 383–392.

Ware, J.E. Jr. & Sherbourne, C.D. (1992). The MOS 36-item short-form health suney (SF-36). 1. Conceptual framework and item selection. Med Care, 30, 473–483.

Wessely, S. & Powell, R. (1989). Fatigue syndromes: a comparison of chronic postviral fatigue with neuromuscular and affective disorders. J Neurol Neurosurg Psychiatry, 52, 940–948.

3

THE CHRONIC FATIGUE SYNDROME

An Update on Important Issues

Irving E. Salit*

Division of Infectious Diseases
The Toronto Hospital
Toronto, Ontario, Canada

ABSTRACT

The Chronic Fatigue Syndrome is a chronic debilitating illness associated with severe fatigue as well as a variety of other complaints. CFS is often considered to be postinfectious and many etiologic agents have been suggested but no consistent infecting agent has been found. Other theories of causation abound but none is clearly favoured by the scientific evidence. Numerous studies confirm the presence of depressive and anxiety syndromes during or even preceding the onset of CFS. Routine blood tests are generally normal but a variety of inconsistent immunologic abnormalities are reported. Cognitive dysfunction is frequently subjectively reported but difficult to

* Address for Correspondence: Dr. Irving E. Salit: Division of Infectious Diseases, The Toronto Hospital, General Division, 200 Elizabeth Street, Eaton North, G-216, Toronto, Ontario, Canada, M5G 2C4. Tel. No. (416) 340-3697; Fax No. (416) 348-8702.

Chronic Fatigue Syndrome, edited by Yehuda and Mostofsky
Plenum Press, New York, 1997

confirm objectively. Many treatments have been reportedly useful in CFS but none is consistently effective. Cognitive behavioural treatment has demonstrated excellent results. Full recovery is very unusual but many subjects improve over time. CFS overlaps with other conditions such as fibromyalgia and depression. The information amongst the general public and popular press differs from that in the scientific literature; there is a need for education of physicians, patients and patient groups with respect to current scientific evidence. CFS is an often misunderstood illness and is a credible area for research.

INTRODUCTION

The Chronic Fatigue Syndrome (CFS) is a chronic debilitating illness associated with severe fatigue (typically exacerbated by exertion) as well as a variety of other complaints including myalgias, subjective cognitive impairment, depressive symptoms, sleep disturbances and headaches (Salit, 1985; Salit, 1995; Salit, 1996a). The illness is defined by symptoms and there are no diagnostic physical findings or laboratory tests. Although the term CFS was first used in 1988 (Holmes), the illness is not new; patients who were diagnosed as neurasthenia a century ago had identical symptoms to those who in later years were diagnosed as having Effort Syndrome, chronic brucellosis or chronic Epstein-Barr virus infection. Although other terms have been used for this condition, such as myalgic encephalomyelitis (ME), Chronic Fatigue and Immune Dysfunction Syndrome (CFIDS) and post-viral fatigue syndrome, CFS is the preferred designation since it is descriptive and operationally defined. There have been utbreaks of illnesses which are quite similar to CFS and which have been called ME or others have been named for the location (eg, Royal Free Disease). The relationship of outbreaks of CFS-like illness to the more common sporadic form of CFS is uncertain. Except where designated, I will be discussing the sporadic form of CFS.

CFS occurs predominantly in women in their 30's and 40's and, although patients are often ill for years, progressive deterioration is very unusual and most subjects at least have some improvement over time. The multisystemic manifestations of CFS have resulted in the involvement of health care professionals and researchers from many different disciplines and the conclusions derived from these disparate approaches have at times been contradictory and confusing. Furthermore, abnormalities are frequently found during the course of clinical investigations in CFS which may be of uncertain relevance to the pathogenesis of the condition. There are currently over 900 published articles on CFS; it is obvious that not all of these publications can be reviewed in the discussions which follow. I will attempt to review some of the salient aspects of CFS and try to put some of the information in perspective.

PRECIPITATING FACTORS

A common thread in the scientific literature and the lay press is that CFS is a postinfectious and especially a postviral condition. In my own studies (Salit, 1996) and those reported by MacDonald (1996), CFS started with an apparent infectious illness in 72% of the subjects. A respiratory illness occurred in 44%, gastrointestinal illness in 9% and both presentations occurred in 47% (MacDonald, 1996). Stressful events in the year prior to onset of CFS were significant in one study (Salit, 1996) but not in another (MacDonald, 1996). Other relevant preceding factors were the increased use of exercise in CFS subjects and they were more frequently nulliparous; factors which were not found to be relevant have included the presence of allergies, contact with animals, smoking, consumption of raw milk or raw meat and foreign travel (MacDonald, 1996). Immunization was not a significant precipitant (Salit, 1996). Most studies have found higher rates of depression prior to the onset of CFS.

Despite the history of an infectious episode at the onset of CFS, one large prospective study followed subjects
who either had or did not have symptomatic infections;
there was no general increase in fatigue in the subjects
who had the infectious illnesses; however, those who did
have a past history of fatigue and psychiatric morbidity
were more likely to develop chronic fatigue (Wessely,
1995).

Numerous infective agents have been implicated as
the cause of CFS; these include the Epstein-Barr Virus,
enteroviruses, human herpesvirus-6 (HHV-6), retroviruses,
etc. (Salit, 1996; Salit, 1996a). Brucellosis was a fashionable cause of chronic fatigue about 50 years ago (Evans,
1947) but has not been associated with CFS more recently.
Recently a stealth virus has been transmitted from a CFS
patient to cats and caused encephalopathy (Martin, 1995).
Although antibody levels to VCA of the Epstein-Barr Virus
may be elevated in CFS, there is no evidence for an excess
replication of EBV in this condition (Swanink, 1995). Similarly, although antibody levels may be elevated to Coxsackie B1 and B4, most studies have been unable to
clearly link enteroviruses to CFS (Swanink, 1994). One
study did suggest that there may be a distinct novel enterovirus which may not be determined by usual serologic
testing (Galbraith, 1995). In one outbreak of CFS in Incline
Village in Lake Tahoe, CFS cases more commonly had active replication of HHV-6 compared to controls (Buchwald,
1992). Although, there is generally no serologic evidence
for HHV-6 as a cause of CFS, HHV-6 variant A may be
more frequently found in CFS than in the general population (Di Luca, 1995). Similarly, HHV-7, hepatitis C and
HSV-1 and HSV-2 are not common precipitants of CFS
(Manian, 1994; Di Luca, 1995; Dale, 1991). Occasional
cases of CFS do occur after Lyme disease and 34% of subjects with Lyme disease do have long-term sequelae which
often include fatigue and fibromyalgia (Dinerman, 1992);
however, during investigations of CFS, Lyme disease is
very rarely found to be the cause (Salit, 1996). Borna disease virus (BDV) has been associated with approximately

one third of Japanese cases of CFS (Nakaya, 1996) but this was not confirmed for German cases of CFS (Bode, 1992).

Although it is clear that there is no defined single infective agent which is associated with the bulk of cases of CFS, there are certainly reports of CFS occurring after many different but definite infections (Salit, 1996); for example, Imboden (1961) found that there could be continued illness with chronic fatigue after influenza and psychological vulnerability predicted this delayed recovery.

Other noninfectious precipitants have been described as being associated with the onset of CFS; these include trauma, allergies and surgery and in some cases there is no apparent precipitating event (Salit, 1996).

There is no lack of theories as to the causation of CFS and these include "chronic candidiasis" (Cater, 1990), airborne microbial contamination especially with Gram negative bacilli and perhaps endotoxin (Teeuw, 1994), excessive levels of chlorinated hydrocarbons (Dunstan, 1995) and sick building syndrome (Chester, 1994). Recently, neurally mediated hypotension (NMH) was described as occurring in 22/23 subjects with CFS and 9/22 had a complete or nearly complete response of their symptoms to therapy for NMH (Bou-Holaigah, 1995). This, however, remains controversial and must be replicated.

In summary, many different infectious and noninfectious illnesses have been described as being associated with the onset of CFS. There is no single infection which has been associated with most cases and it seems most unlikely that any single infection causes the majority of cases of CFS. The infections that have resulted in CFS, cause CFS only rarely so one must be dealing with an unusual variant of an infective agent or, much more likely, the patient who develops CFS must have some predisposition. The lack of clusters of CFS occurring within families make a mutant virus quite unlikely. Another possibility is that precipitating factors can trigger immunologic or physiologic changes which then result in the reactivation of an existing virus such as HHV-6 (Josephs, 1991). There is a general consensus amongst investigators that a multi-factorial theory of causation is most plausible (Salit, 1996a).

PSYCHOLOGICAL FACTORS

Patients who present with the symptom of chronic fatigue (and not necessarily CFS) frequently have psychiatric disorders including depression (Manu, 1989). Some of the psychiatric disorders frequently associated with chronic fatigue include affective disorders, anxiety, somatization disorders and panic disorders. Studies that have included a systematic assessment of the mental state of subjects with CFS have found that many also have psychological distress. Numerous studies have confirmed that a substantial proportion meet the criteria for depressive and anxiety syndromes with high rates of depression during CFS and even preceding the onset of CFS (Taerk, 1987; Kruesi, 1989; Sharpe, 1992; Katon, 1991). The severity of depressive symptoms are usually found to be intermediate between that seen in major depression and that seen in comparative physical disorders which are also associated with fatigue (Wessely, 1989). These studies do seem to indicate that the depression seen in CFS is out of proportion to that which can be explained by the disabling fatigue itself. Because of the above findings, a systematic psychosocial history and mental state examination should be done on all patients including an assessment of mood and risk of suicide (Salit, 1996a). It is important to note that the most current and commonly used case definition of CFS does not exclude subjects with major depression (Fukuda, 1994).

A major subject of contention is whether the psychological disorders associated with CFS actually precede or lead to CFS as opposed to being a consequence of the other symptoms of CFS (such as fatigue and disability). A number of studies have found that "emotionality" (Blakely, 1991) and psychologic disorders (Wessely, 1995) are predisposing factors for CFS. Studies on the psychological aspects of CFS should, therefore, include appropriate controls who have similar fatigue and disability. Several studies have compared CFS to subjects with neurologic disorders such as multiple sclerosis (MS). Patients with CFS generally have significantly more severe depressive symptoms compared with patients with MS and healthy controls and they have a greater lifetime prevalence of depression and dysthymia compared to MS subjects (Krupp, 1994; Pepper, 1993). Both CFS and depressed subjects endorse a higher percentage of somatization disorder symptoms than either multiple sclerosis or healthy control groups but very few meet the strict DSM-III-R criteria for somatization disorder (Johnson, 1996).

Some subsets of patients with CFS may have even higher rates of psychiatric morbidity; these would include subjects with apparent sensitivities to chemicals and those who have no clear date of onset of the CFS (Fiedler, 1996). Subjects with CFS tend to attribute their symptoms to external causes (such as a virus) whereas a comparative depressed group experience inward attribution (Powell, 1990). Children with the Chronic Fatigue Syndrome also have high rates of depression and poor social adjustment (Walford, 1993). The epidemic form of CFS has generally not been rigorously studied from the point of view of psychologic disorders. The Royal Free epidemic, however, was later thought to be an episode of "mass hysteria" and a case-control follow-up study of nurses involved in the epidemic was done by McEvedy and Beard (1973). They found that the affected nurses when compared with matched controls had higher neuroticism scores, had more illness prior to the epidemic and that subsequent to the epidemic had more psychiatric difficulties. Subjects with CFS but without a psychiatric disorder tend to have less severe illness than those with an associated psychiatric disorder (Shanks, 1995).

Antidepressants seem to be helpful in improving sleep and reducing pain particularly in CFS patients who also meet the criteria for fibromyalgia (Lynch, 1991; Goodnick,

1992) but there was no benefit in one placebo-controlled trial (Vercoulen, 1996a). Patients with CFS often report a very heightened sensitivity to medication so many are unable to tolerate even small doses of antidepressants. Cognitive-behavioural therapies have been used (Sharpe, 1993; Butler, 1991; Friedberg, 1995) and this approach seems to be logical; however, a brief form of this approach was not shown to be effective in one randomized clinical trial (Lloyd, 1993). A subsequent randomized controlled trial did indicate considerable benefit of this approach in CFS (Sharpe, 1996).

In summary, many studies on subjects with CFS have found a high prevalence of psychologic distress. How are the psychological disorders and CFS related? The fatigue, psychological problems and other symptoms may be an intrinsic part of CFS and all are precipitated and continue because of the same factors. An alternative explanation is that the psychological problems occur as a result of the physical dysfunction seen in CFS; this would indicate that there is more than one biologic process which is operative. Lastly, one has to consider whether there is a psychologic predisposition to CFS. For example, this could occur by increasing the susceptibility to infections or by allowing the symptoms of an infection to persist much longer than they otherwise would. Fatigue seems to occur on a continuum in the general population and CFS is one extreme of that continuum (Pawlikowska, 1994). It is clear that psychiatric disorders seem to occur at a high rate in subjects who have chronic fatigue and these disorders seem to be an explanation for the chronic fatigue; if that is the case, then why can not more severe forms of chronic fatigue such as CFS also be explained on the same basis?

TEST ABNORMALITIES

Routine blood tests are generally normal including complete blood count, sedimentation rate and tests of hepatic, renal and thyroid function. I have commonly noted, however, elevations of IgG and/or IgM, an elevation of the CD_4/CD_8 ratio and an elevated 2–5A oligoadenylate synthetase. In one study, in comparison to healthy controls, subjects with CFS also had significant elevations in immune complexes, IgG, alkaline phosphatase, cholesterol, atypical lymphocytes and there was a lower lactic dehydrogenase (Bates, 1995). CFS is often associated with allergy and eosinophil cationic protein serum levels were significantly higher in CFS patients compared to controls (Conti, 1996). Insulin-like growth factor-I (Somatomedin C) levels were not found to be elevated in CFS unlike subjects with fibromyalgia (Buchwald, 1996). These tests could be included in research studies but should not be considered part of routine investigations. Fukuda (1994) has recommended that only a minimum battery of laboratory screening tests should be done and these might include a complete blood count with differential; erythrocyte sedimentation rate; hepatic transaminases, total protein, albumin, globulin, alkaline phosphatase, calcium, phophorus, glucose, electrolytes, urea nitrogen, creatinine, thyroid stimulating hormone and urinalysis. Routinely doing other screening tests for all patients has no known value. However, further tests should be to exclude specific diagnoses which might be suggested by particular symptoms in an individual patient.

Immunologic abnormalities are not consistent between studies and are only found in a minority of subjects with CFS. Alterations of lymphocyte subsets have been described as well as decreased natural killer cell function (Landay, 1991; Klimas, 1990). Similarly, studies on interleukins have also not shown uniform results (Rasmussen, 1994; MacDonald, 1996). Lymphocyte phenotypes are quite variable; Strauss (1993) noted reduced proportions of CD_4 cells bearing CD_{45} surface antigen, increased levels of various adhesion molecules and reduced responses when lymphocytes were stimulated with mitogens or superantigen. Landay (1991) found reduced CD_{11b}, increased CD_{38} and increased HLA-DR. These changes increased as the disease was more severe and seemed to get better over time with clinical improvement. Swanink (1996) found a decrease in the expression of CD_{11b} on CD_8 cells but did not find an increased expression of CD_{38} and HLA-DR; circulating cytokines were normal. An important finding in this study was that the immunologic test results did not correlate with fatigue severity or psychologic well being.

CT brain scans are normal but brain abnormalities have been noted using MRI and SPECT scanning (Ichise, 1992; Natelson, 1993). Compared with normal controls, CFS subjects have significantly lower cortical/cerebellar regional cerebral blood flow ratios throughout multiple brain regions (Ichise, 1992). Subjects with major depression may also have decreased cortical and subcortical regional cerebral blood flow (O'Connell, 1989). The MRI abnormalities have not generally been confirmed in CFS (Cope, 1996).

Sleep disturbances are very frequent and can be documented in objective sleep studies but the nature of the abnormalities is quite variable (Whelton, 1988; Krupp , 1993). Most patients with CFS describe unrefreshing sleep and show a prominent alpha electroencephalographic, nonrapid eye movement sleep anomaly similar to that seen in fibromyalgia (Whelton, 1992).

Standardized psychological testing has documented a variety of disturbances including depression and increased stress (Taerk, 1987; Pawlikowska, 1994). Cognitive dysfunction is a frequent complaint yet objective testing does not consistently demonstrate this abnormality (Altay, 1990); there are also no gross deficits in either perceptual, attentional or short-term memory processes throughout prolonged challenge (Scheffers, 1992). One study did find that subjects with CFS had difficulty on tasks that require simultaneous processing of complex cognitive information (DeLuca, 1993).

Muscle abnormalities have generally been noted to be minor or nonexistent (Lloyd, 1988; Stokes, 1988).

In summary, routine blood tests are useful to do in the investigation of CFS in order to rule out other disorders which could be a cause of the fatigue. Other detailed testing often shows variable results and cannot be used to specifically diagnose CFS. It still remains to be determined if there are any clearcut differences in the frequency of the above abnormalities in CFS compared to other conditions such as chronic fatigue, fibromyalgia and psychiatric disorders such as depression. Any studies on the apparent test abnormalities should always include comparisons with appropriate controls. It would be important to know if the observed changes noted above result from an integral part of the pathophysiology of CFS or whether they are epiphenomena. For example, some abnormalities may arise as a result of forced disruptions of the patient's usual lifestyle, psychosocial distress or deconditioning.

MANAGEMENT AND OUTCOME

Different therapies have been reported to be beneficial in CFS but these have either not been confirmed or have been refuted (Straus, 1991; Cox, 1991; Behan, 1990; Bou-Holaigah, 1995). Although reportedly beneficial, efamol, magnesium and immunoglobulin injections are not routinely used in clinical practice in part because the experience of the patients and the physicians is that they are not reliably useful. There is ample experience with patients who have attributed improvement to something that they have tried (such as an alternative treatment) but there is generally improvement over time irrespective of what therapy the patient may have tried. Many physicians try low doses of antidepressants which may cause some improvement in sleep and myalgias. Many patients with CFS often report a heightened sensitivity to medication so treatment should be started at the lowest dose before gradually escalating the dosage. One randomized double-blind placebo-controlled study of fluoxetine found no beneficial effects on any characteristic of CFS (Vercoulen, 1996a). Other ineffective treatments include acyclovir (Strauss, 1988), leukocyte extract (Lloyd, 1993) and B_{12}-folic acid-liver extract (Kaslow, 1989). Despite the prevalence of a history of atopy, a trial of terfenadine was not found to be beneficial

(Steinberg, 1996). Essential fatty acids (Behan, 1990) and Ampligen or poly (I):poly (C_{12} U) (Strayer, 1994) have been reported to produce some improvement in symptoms although these trials have not been replicated. Alternative and complementary therapies and dietary regimens are widely used by patients with CFS although their efficacy is largely unevaluated.

Many subjects indicate that the bulk of their improvement comes from a clear understanding of their condition and from suggestions for subsequent management; these would include avoiding expensive unproven therapies, participating in a graded exercise program, being aware that they do not have a contagious illness and having an understanding of the multifactorial aspects of the condition. Patients should be prepared to accept treatment for their major symptoms such as the sleep abnormalities and depression. The family physician should provide the bulk of care for subjects with CFS; multiple visits to subspecialists is often not beneficial especially if patients are searching for a simple and easily reversible cause for their symptoms.

There has been some interest in the use of cognitive behavioural treatment for the Chronic Fatigue Syndrome. A brief form of this approach was not shown to be effective in a randomized controlled trial (Lloyd, 1993) but two recent studies have indicated that this approach may be beneficial. Friedberg (1995) showed a trend towards reduced depression-symptoms scores and, in the most depressed patients, there was improvement in stress, fatigue severity and fatigue-related thinking. It was suggested that depression in CFS was mediated by maladaptive thinking. In a randomized control trial, cognitive behavioural therapy was found to be well accepted by the patients and 73% achieved a satisfactory outcome compared to only 20% of subjects who were given only medical care (Sharpe, 1996). The improvement in disability continued after completion of therapy. In this study, illness beliefs and coping behaviour which have been associated with a poor outcome changed more with cognitive behaviour therapy than with the medical care alone.

There is increasing evidence as to the prognosis of CFS. Studies in tertiary care settings indicate that while many patients with CFS do improve, few report complete recovery at two to three years after diagnosis (Sharpe, 1992; Wilson, 1994); very few patients show significant deterioration over time and the condition is not fatal. Functional status and outcome appear to be better in patients who are identified in community and primary care studies compared to tertiary care settings (Buchwald, 1995). I have found that subjects who have an acute onset to their illness have better rates of recovery than those with a gradual onset (Salit, 1996). Outcomes are also worse in those who have a fixed belief about a viral causation to their illness and in those who belong to community support groups (Wilson, 1994; Sharpe, 1992). In one prospective study, the following factors were predictors of improvement: a subjective sense of control over symptoms, less fatigue, shorter duration of complaints and a relative absence of physical attributions (Vercoulen, 1996). Treatment by specialists and alternative practitioners did not predict improvement. Psychological well being also did not predict improvement in this study; others have suggested that this factor does play a part in the perpetuation of complaints and Sharpe et al. (1992) found a relation between depression and improvement. Avoidance of physical activity is also thought to play a part in the continuation of the symptoms (Butler, 1991).

After 4–5 years of illness approximately 3% of subjects have fully recovered and an additional 17–50% have improved (Vercoulen, 1996; Clark, 1995; Salit, unpublished data; Wilson, 1994). Only 2% of subjects develop another medical diagnosis to explain their fatigue whereas in about 20% an alternative psychiatric diagnosis was felt likely (Wilson, 1994).

In summary, patients with CFS should be reassured about the generally positive outcome of their illness; however, many patients may suffer persistent disability, especially those with certain fixed beliefs about CFS and those with persistent psychiatric disorders. Although the impact of treatment on the natural history is unknown, there is suggestive evidence that multidisciplinary rehabilitative approaches and active treatment of psychiatric disorders, perhaps using a cognitive-behavioural approach, are likely to improve the outcome (Sharpe, 1996; Salit, 1996a). Management should include the provision of accurate and balanced information. Costly and ineffective alternative therapies should be avoided.

DELINEATING CFS FROM OTHER CONDITIONS

CFS overlaps to a great extent with fibromyalgia and major depression (Goldenberg, 1990; Taerk, 1987; Kruesi, 1989; Behan, 1990). Patients with CFS should be evaluated for these latter conditions as well. Since there is no diagnostic test for CFS, a definitive diagnosis is not possible. If patients with CFS do meet the case definition for that condition it does not preclude a further diagnosis such as fibromyalgia or major depression (Fukuda, 1994).

The case definitions of CFS can reasonably define a syndrome but they do not differentiate CFS from other condition such as fibromyalgia. A new case definition for CFS is less restrictive with respect to the requirement for physical findings since these are quite infrequent (Fukuda, 1994). It would be useful to subdivide cases of CFS based on associated conditions such as depression, other psychiatric disorders, significant sleep disorders and fibromyalgia. Researchers in CFS and fibromyalgia have published position papers on those conditions (Salit, 1996; Wolfe, 1996) and their assessments of the respective conditions indicate a remarkable similarity between fibromyalgia and CFS.

ASSESSMENT FOR INSURANCE PURPOSES

Because of the severe disabling fatigue, many subjects with CFS are unable to work on a full-time basis. The insurance assessment should be considered an integral part of the management of patients with CFS.

The aim should be for the patient to remain in the workplace or return to the workplace whenever possible. Assessments should be based on the symptoms and degree of disability and not on fulfilment of any diagnostic criteria for CFS (Salit, 1996a). The test results are useful for research purposes and to exclude other conditions; they are not useful in accepting or neglecting a patient for disability benefits.

COMMUNITY AND PROFESSIONAL INTERACTIONS

The academic medical community, on the one hand, and the general public and popular press, on the other hand, differ in their perceptions with regard to CFS (MacLean, 1994). Patients often rely upon books, newspapers, magazines and community groups for information about CFS. Some of that information is at variance with the current body of scientific information. For example, the lay press often has information on the latest virus which is the apparent cause of CFS, there are claims of "miracle cures" or there is a focus on management strategies which clearly differs from currently suggested approaches by the professional community. Although initial scientific studies did focus on a persistent virus as an etiologic agent, subsequent studies have not supported the concept of a single infecting agent that is the cause of CFS. This, however, remains the dominant model amongst the public and press. Any model which incorporates stressors and psychosocial aspects of CFS is often greeted with hostility. Alternative explanations for which inadequate scientific evidence exists includes environmental hypersensitivity, severe immunodeficiency and yeast overgrowth. Current evidence suggests that there are multiple interactive biologic and psychosocial factors that contribute to the clinical expression of CFS.

Many physicians do not have an appropriate understanding of the patients' symptoms which may be regarded as "nothing" if there is no physical condition to explain those symptoms. Patients' symptoms are often not taken seriously if it is felt by the physician that they may be at least in part psychologically based. Patients with CFS often come to the physician for a validation of their symptoms but may be met with skepticism, lack of acceptance and a lack of compassion. The doctor-patient relationship may be strained by the dichotomization of illness into physical or emotional and by the patient's denial of the role of psychosocial distress.

Physicians should not dismiss the symptoms of CFS as trivial since the illness has a major impact on patients and may cause severe disability. There is obviously a need for education of physicians, patients and patient groups with respect to the current evidence gleaned from scientific studies. CFS is a credible area of research; hopefully such research will continue. Health care professionals and those with CFS have to accept the body of scientific evidence and move forward to use that information to improve the lives of patients.

ACKNOWLEDGMENT

The author thanks Shirley Magnaye for excellent assistance in the preparation of this chapter.

REFERENCES

1. Altay HT, Toner BB, Brooker H, Abbey SE, Salit IE, Garfinkel PE: The neuropsychological dimensions of postinfectious neuromyasthenia (chronic fatigue syndrome): a preliminary report. Int J Psychiat Med 1990; 20 (2):141–149.
2. Bates DW, Buchwald D, Lee J, et al: Clinical laboratory test findings in patients with chronic fatigue syndrome. Arch Intern Med 1995; 155: 97–103.
3. Behan PO, Behan WMH, Horrobin DF: Effect of high doses of essential fatty acids on the postviral fatigue syndrome. Acta Neurol Scand 1990; 82: 209–216.

4. Blakely AA, Howard RC, Sosich RM, et al: Psychiatric symptoms, personality and ways of coping in chronic fatigue syndrome. Psychol Med 1991; 21: 347–362.

5. Bode L, Komaroff AL, Ludwig H: No serologic evidence of borna disease virus in patients with chronic fatigue syndrome (letter). Clin Infect Dis 1992; 15: 1049.

6. Bou-Holaigah I, Rowe PC, Kan J, Calkins H: The relationship between neurally mediated hypotension and the chronic fatigue syndrome. JAMA 1995; 274: 961–967.

7. Buchwald D, Cheney PR, Peterson DL, et al: A chronic illness characterized by fatigue, neurologic and immunologic disorders, and active Human Herpesvirus Type 6 infection. Ann Intern Med 1992; 116:103–113.

8. Buchwald D, Umali P, Umali J, et al: Chronic fatigue and the Chronic Fatigue Syndrome: Prevalence in a Pacific Northwest Health Care System. Ann Intern Med 1995; 123(2): 81–88.

9. Buchwald D, Umali J, Stene M: Insulin-like growth factor-I (Somatomedin C) levels in chronic fatigue syndrome and fibromyalgia. J Rheum 1996; 23: 739–742.

10. Butler S, Chalder T, Ron M, Wessely S: Cognitive behaviour therapy in chronic fatigue syndrome. J Neurol Neurosurg Psychiat 1991; 54: 153–158.

11. Cater RE: Chronic intestinal candidiasis as a possible etiological factor in the chronic fatigue syndrome. Medical Hypotheses 1995; 44: 507–515.

12. Chester AC, Levine PH: Concurrent sick building syndrome and chronic fatigue syndrome: epidemic neuromyasthenia revisited. Clin Infect Dis 1994; 18(Suppl 1): S43-S48.

13. Clark MR, Katon W, Russo J, et al: Chronic fatigue: risk factors for symptom persistence in a 21-year follow-up study. Am J Med 1995; 98: 187–195.

14. Conti F, Magrini L, Priori R, et al: Eosinophil cationic protein serum levels and allergy in chronic fatigue syndrome. Allergy 1996; 51: 124–127.

15. Cope H, David AS: Neuroimaging in chronic fatigue syndrome. J Neurol Neurosurg Psychiat 1996; 60: 471–473.

16. Cox IM, Campbell MJ, Dowson D: Red blood cell magnesium and chronic fatigue syndrome. Lancet 1991; 337: 757–760.

17. Dale JK, Di Bisceglie AM, Hofnagle JH, Straus SE: Chronic fatigue syndrome: lack of association with hepatitis C virus infection. J Med Virol 1991; 34: 119–121.

18. DeLuca J, Johnson SK, Natelson BH: Information processing efficiency in chronic fatigue syndrome and multiple sclerosis. Arch Neurol 1993; 50: 301–304.

19. Di Luca D, Zorzenon M, Mirandola P, et al: Human Herpesvirus 6 and Human Herpesvirus 7 in chronic fatigue syndrome. J Clin Microbiol 1995; 33: 1660–1661.
20. Dinerman, H, Steere AC: Lyme disease associated with fibromyalgia. Ann Intern Med 1992; 117:281–285.
21. Dunstan RH, Donohoe M, Taylor W, et al: A preliminary investigation of chlorinated hydrocarbons and chronic fatigue syndrome. Med J Aust 1995; 163: 294–297.
22. Evans AC: Brucellosis in the United States. Am J Public Health 1947; 37: 139–151.
23. Fiedler N, Kipen HM, DeLuca J, et al: A controlled comparison of multiple chemical sensitivities and chronic fatigue syndrome. Psychosom Med 1996; 58:38–49.
24. Friedberg F, Krupp LB: A comparison of cognitive behavioural treatment for chronic fatigue syndrome and primary depression. Clin Infect Dis 1995; 20: 717–718.
25. Fukuda K, Straus SE, Hickie I, et al: The Chronic Fatigue Syndrome: a comprehensive approach to its definition and study. Ann Intern Med 1994; 121: 953–959.
26. Galbraith DN, Nairn C, Clements GB: Phylogenetic analysis of short enteroviral sequences from patients with chronic fatigue syndrome. J General Virol 1995; 76: 1701–1707.
27. Gold D, Bowden R, Sixbey J, et al: Chronic Fatigue: A prospective clinical and virologic study. JAMA 1990; 264:48–53.
28. Goldenberg DL, Simms RW, Geiger A, Komaroff AL: High frequency of fibromyalgia in patients with chronic fatigue seen in a primary care practice. Arthritis Rheum 1990; 33: 381–387.
29. Goodnick PJ, Sandoval R, Brickman A, Klimas NG: Bupropion treatment of fluoxetine-resistant chronic fatigue syndrome. Biol Psychiat 1992; 32: 834–838.
30. Holmes GP, Kaplan J, Grantz N, et al: Chronic Fatigue Syndrome: a working case definition. Ann Intern Med 1988; 108: 387–389.
31. Ichise M, Salit IE, Abbey SE, et al: Assessment of regional cerebral perfusion by 99Tcm-HMPAO SPECT in chronic fatigue syndrome. Nucl Med Commun 1992; 13: 767–772.
32. Imboden J, Canter A, Cluff L: Convalescence from influenza: a study of the psychological and clinical determinants. Arch Intern Med 1961; 108:393–399.
33. Johnson SK, DeLuca J, Natelson BH: Assessing somatization disorder in the chronic fatigue syndrome. Psychosom Med 1996; 58: 50–57.
34. Josephs SF, Henry BE, Balachandran N, et al: HHV-6 reactivation in chronic fatigue syndrome. Lancet 1991; 337: 1346–1347.
35. Kaslow JE, Rucker L, Onishi R: Liver extract-folic acid-cyanocobalamin vs placebo for chronic fatigue syndrome. Arch Intern Med 1989; 149: 2501–2503.

36. Katon WJ, Buchwald D, Simon GE, Russo J, Mease P: Psychiatric illness in patients with chronic fatigue and rheumatoid arthritis. J Gen Intern Med 1991; 6: 277–285.
37. Klimas NG, Salvato FR, Morgan R, Fletcher MA: Immunologic abnormalities in chronic fatigue syndrome. J Clin Microbiol 1990; 28: 1403–1410.
38. Kruesi MJP, Dale JK, Straus SE: Psychiatric diagnoses in patients who have chronic fatigue syndrome. J Clin Psychiat 1989; 50: 53–56.
39. Krupp LB, Jandorf L, Coyle PK, Mendelson WB: Sleep disturbance in chronic fatigue syndrome. J Psychosom Res 1993; 37: 325–331.
40. Krupp LB, Sliwinski M, Masur DM, et al: Cognitive functioning and depression in patients with chronic fatigue syndrome and multiple sclerosis. Arch Neurol 1994; 51: 705–710.
41. Landay AL, Jessop C, Lennette ET, Levy JA: Chronic fatigue syndrome: clinical condition associated with immune activation. Lancet 1991; 338: 707–712.
42. Lloyd AR, Hales JP, Gandevia SC: Muscle strength,endurance and recovery in the post infection fatigue syndrome. J Neurol Neurosurg Psychiat 1988; 51: 1316–1322.
43. Lloyd AR, Hickie I, Brockman A, et al: Immunologic and psychologic therapy for patients with chronic fatigue syndrome: a double-blind, placebo-controlled trial. Am J Med 1993; 94: 197–203.
44. Lynch S, Seth R, Montgomery S: Antidepressant therapy in the chronic fatigue syndrome.. Brit J Gen Pract 1991; 41: 339–342.
45. MacDonald KL, Osterholm MT, LeDell KH, et al: A case-control study to assess possible triggers and cofactors in Chronic Fatigue Syndrome. Am J Med 1996; 100:548–554.
46. MacLean G, Wessely S: Professional and popular views of chronic fatigue syndrome. BMJ 1994; 308: 776–777.
47. Manian FA: Simultaneous measurement of antibodies to Epstein-Barr virus, Human Herpesvirus 6, Herpes Simplex virus types 1 and 2, and 14 enteroviruses in chronic fatigue syndrome: is there evidence of activation of a nonspecific polyclonal immune response? Clin Infect Dis 1994; 19: 448–453.
48. Manu P, Matthews DA, Lane TJ, et al: Depression among patients with a chief complaint of chronic fatigue.. J Affective Disord 1989; 17: 165–172.
49. Martin WJ, Glass RT: Acute encephalopathy induced in cats with a stealth virus isolated from a patient with chronic fatigue syndrome. Pathobiol 1995; 63: 115–118.
50. McEvedy CP, Beard AW: A controlled follow-up of cases involved in an epidemic of "benign myalgic encephalomyelitis". Brit J Psychiat 1973; 122: 141–150.

51. Miller NA, Carmichael HA, Calder BD, et al: Antibody to coxsackie B virus in diagnosing postviral fatigue syndrome. BMJ 1991; 302: 140–143.

52. Nakaya T, Takahashi H, Nakamura Y, et al: Demonstration of borna disease virus RNA in peripheral blood mononuclear cells derived from Japanese patients with chronic fatigue syndrome. FEBS Letters 1996; 378: 145–149.

53. Natelson BH, Cohen JM, Brassloff I, Lee H: A controlled study of brain magnetic resonance imaging in patients with the chronic fatigue syndrome. J Neurol Sci 1993; 120: 213–217.

54. O'Connell RA, Van Heertum RL, Billick SB, et al: Single photon emission computed tomography (SPECT) with [^{123}I]IMP in the differential diagnosis of psychiatric disorders. J Neuropsych 1989; 1: 145–153.

55. Pawlikowska T, Chalder T, Hirsch S, et al: A population based study of fatigue and psychological distress. BMJ 1994; 308: 763–766.

56. Peel M: Rehabilitation in Postviral syndrome. J Soc Occup Med 1988; 38: 44–45.

57. Pepper CM, Krupp LB, Friedberg F, et al: A comparison of neuropsychiatric characteristics in chronic fatigue syndrome, multiple sclerosis, and major depression. J Neuropsych Clin Neurosci 1993; 5: 200–205.

58. Powell R, Dolan R, Wessely S: Attributions and self-esteem in depression and chronic fatigue syndromes. J Psychosom Res 1990; 34: 665–673.

59. Prasher D, Smith A, Findley L: Sensory and cognitive event-related potentials in myalgic encephalomyelitis. J Neurol Neurosurg Psychiat 1990; 53(3): 247–53.

60. Rasmussen AK, Nielsen H, Andersen V, et al: Chronic fatigue syndrome -- a controlled cross sectional study. J Rheum 1994; 21: 1527–1531.

61. Salit, I.E: Sporadic postinfective neuromyasthenia: persistent illness after acute infections. Can Med Ass J 1985; 133:659–663.

62. Salit IE: The chronic fatigue syndrome: an overview of important issues. J Musculoskeletal Pain 1995; 3: 17–24.

63. Salit IE: Precipitating factors for the chronic fatigue syndrome. J Psych Res 1996 (in press).

64. Salit IE, The Vancouver Chronic Fatigue Syndrome Consensus Group: The chronic fatigue syndrome: a position paper. J Rheum 1996a; 23: 540–544.

65. Scheffers MK, Johnson R, Grafman J, et al: Attention and short-term memory in chronic fatigue syndrome patients: an event-related potential analysis. Neurol 1992; 42: 1667–1675.

66. Shanks MF, Ho-Yen DO: A clinical study of chronic fatigue syndrome. Brit J Psych 1995; 166: 798–801.

67. Sharpe MC, Hawton KE, Seagraott V, Pasvol G: Patients who present with fatigue: a follow up of referrals to an infectious diseases clinic.. BMJ 1992; 305: 147–152.
68. Sharpe M, Hawton K, Simkin S, et al: Cognitive behaviour therapy for the chronic fatigue syndrome: a randomized controlled trial. BMJ 1996; 312: 22–26.
69. Steinberg P, McNutt BE, Marshall P, et al: Double-blind placebo-controlled study of the efficacy of oral terfenadine in the treatment of chronic fatigue syndrome. J Allergy Clin Immunol 1996; 97: 119–126.
70. Stokes MJ, Cooper RG, Edwards RHT: Normal muscle strength and fatiguability in patients with effort syndromes. BMJ 1988; 297: 1014–1016.
71. Straus SE, Dale JK, Tobi M, et al: Acyclovir treatment of the chronic fatigue syndrome; lack of efficacy in a placebo controlled trial.. N Engl J Med 1988; 319: 1692–1698.
72. Straus SE: Intravenous immunoglobulin treatment for the chronic fatigue syndrome. Am J Med 1991; 89: 551–552.
73. Straus SE, Fritz S, Dale JK, et al: Lymphocyte phenotype and function in the chronic fatigue syndrome. J Clin Immunol 1993; 13: 30–40.
74. Strayer DR, Carter WA, Brodsky I, et al: A controlled clinical trial with a specifically configured RNA drug, poly (I) *mD poly (C12U), in chronic fatigue syndrome. Clin Infect Dis 1994; 18: S88-S95.
75. Swanink CMA, Melchers WJG, van der Meer JWM, et al: Enteroviruses and the chronic fatigue syndrome. Clin Infect Dis 1994; 19: 860–864.
76. Swanink CMA, van der Meer JWM, Vercoulen JHMM, et al: Epstein-Barr virus (EBV) and the chronic fatigue syndrome: normal virus load in blood and normal immunologic reactivity in the EBV regression assay. Clin Infect Dis 1995; 20: 1390–1392.
77. Swanink CM, Vercoulen JH, Galama JM, et al: Lymphocyte subsets, apoptosis, and cytokines in patients with chronic fatigue syndrome. J Infect Dis 1996; 173: 460–463.
78. Taerk GS, Toner BA, Salit IE, et al: Depression in patients with neuromyasthenia (benign myalgic encephalomyelitis). Int J Psychiat Med 1987; 17: 49–56.
79. Teeuw KB, Vandenbroucke-Grauls CMJE, Verhoef J: Airborne gram-negative bacteria and endotoxin in sick building syndrome. Arch Intern Med 1994; 154: 2339–2345.
80. Vercoulen JHMM, Swanink CMA, Fennis JFM, et al: Prognosis in chronic fatigue syndrome: a prospective study on the natural course. J Neurol Neurosurg Psychiat 1996; 60: 489–494.
81. Vercoulen JHMM, Swanink CMA, Zitman FG, et al: Randomised, double-blind, placebo-controlled study of fluoxetine in chronic fatigue syndrome. Lancet 1996a; 347: 858–861.

82. Walford GA, Nelson WMcC, McCluskey DR; Fatigue, depression, and social adjustment in chronic fatigue syndrome. Arch Dis Child 1993; 68: 384–388.

83. Wessely S, Powell R: Fatigue syndromes:a comparison of chronic "postviral" fatigue with neuromuscular and affective disorder. J Neurol Neurosurg Psychiat 1989; 52: 940–948.

84. Wessely S, Chalder T, Hirsch S, et al: Postinfectious fatigue: prospective cohort study in primary care. Lancet 1995; 345: 1333–1338.

85. Whelton C, Saskin P, Salit H, Moldofsky H: Post-viral fatigue syndrome and sleep. Sleep Res 1988; 17: 307.

86. Wilson A, Hickie I, Lloyd A, et al: Longitudinal study of outcome of chronic fatigue syndrome. BMJ 1994; 308: 756–759.

87. Wolfe F, The Vancouver Fibromyalgia Consensus Group: Special report: the fibromyalgia syndrome: a consensus report on fibromyalgia and disability. J Rheum 1996; 23: 534–539.

4

EFFORTS TO REDUCE HETEROGENEITY IN CHRONIC FATIGUE SYNDROME RESEARCH

Christopher Christodoulou,[1,2*] John DeLuca,[1,2,3] Susan K. Johnson,[1,2,3] Gudrun Lange,[1,2,3] and Benjamin H. Natelson[3]

[1]Department of Research
Kessler Institute for Rehabilitation
West Orange, New Jersey
[2]Department of Physical Medicine and
    Rehabilitation
[3]Department of Neurosciences
UMDNJ-New Jersey Medical School
Newark, New Jersey

Individuals with Chronic Fatigue Syndrome (CFS) suffer from persistent, debilitating fatigue, accompanied by a variety of neuropsychiatric, infectious, and rheumatological symptoms. Researchers have not yet discovered the cause of CFS, but a variety of etiologies have been proposed, ranging from viral/immunological (Komaroff,

* Address correspondence to: Christopher Christodoulou, Ph.D., Fatigue Research Center, New Jersey Medical School, 88 Ross St., East Orange, NJ 07018.

Chronic Fatigue Syndrome, edited by Yehuda and Mostofsky
Plenum Press, New York, 1997

1988; Strober, 1994) to psychiatric (Manu, Lane, & Matthews, 1992). As this range of possibilities suggests, arguments exist as to whether CFS is a psychiatric condition resulting from psychological stressors or a nonpsychiatric medical disorder resulting directly from an infectious or toxic agent. Those favoring a psychiatric interpretation have pointed to an increased incidence of affective symptomatology in CFS patient samples (Kruesi, Dale, & Straus, 1989; Lane, Manu, Matthews, 1991). In contrast, those supporting a viral/immunological hypothesis have noted immune system dysregulation (Landay, Jessop, Lennette, & Levy, 1991; Patarca, Klimas, Lugtendorf, Antoni, & Fletcher, 1994) and abnormalities on neuroimaging (Natelson, Cohen, Brassloff, & Lee, 1993) in CFS samples. David (1991) presented three general possibilities as to the role of psychiatric disturbance in CFS. First, psychiatric disturbance could develop as a reaction to the chronic illness associated with CFS; second, CFS could be a misdiagnosed form of psychiatric malady; third, both CFS and psychiatric disorder could result from a common cause.

The psychiatric/non-psychiatric etiological conundrum has been reflected in changes in the CDC definition of CFS. The initial definition excluded all psychiatric illnesses (Holmes, et al., 1988), but later revisions allow inclusion of a variety of affective disorders (Fukuda, et al., 1994; Schluederberg, et al., 1992). The latest international NIH/CDC study group strongly emphasized the need to clarify the role of psychiatric disorders in CFS (Fukuda, et al., 1994). Furthermore, the committee recommended that researchers stratify patient samples according to the presence or absence of coexisting psychiatric conditions. They concluded that there was an essential need to subgroup CFS samples on the basis of such conditions, especially with regard to anxiety and depression. In sum, there is a clear and widespread recognition for the need to reduce CFS sample heterogeneity, particularly as it pertains to psychiatric symptomatology.

1. STRATEGIES FOR REDUCING HETEROGENEITY IN CFS SAMPLES

It is our belief that CFS will eventually be found to be a heterogeneous syndrome arising from a variety of causes. The history of medicine is replete with examples of this occurring for other medical syndromes. Congestive heart failure, for example, produces the same clinical picture regardless of whether the heart disease responsible is caused by diet induced atherosclerosis or viral infection. Our research at the UMDNJ Fatigue Research Center has attempted to identify a more homogeneous group of CFS patients who were previously in good physical and mental health. A hypothesis driving this work is that there is an increased likelihood that these CFS patients resemble those suffering from a physical cause of fatigue, such as multiple sclerosis (MS), as opposed to those whose fatigue is thought to result from a psychiatric disturbance, such as major depression. Our work has addressed the issue of heterogeneity in three ways: first, through the careful selection of CFS patients, second, by the identification of adequate control and comparison patient groups, and finally, through the stratification of CFS samples.

Patients in our more recent studies not only fulfilled the CDC case definition (Holmes, et al., 1988; Schluederberg, et al., 1992), but also met further strict inclusionary criteria. First, our CFS subjects had an absence of psychiatric disorder in the five years prior to CFS onset. This criterion essentially eliminated CFS patients with a prior lifetime history of psychiatric disorder. Second, these CFS subjects had an illness duration of no more than four years. This criterion was included to reduce the likelihood of symptoms that might arise from psychosocial consequences associated with chronic illness. Third, their CFS symptoms were of at least moderate severity at the time of intake, ensuring a level of symptomatology which has had a significant impact upon patients' lives and is most likely to be detected by research measurements. Using these additional criteria to identify potential subjects has served to increase the homogeneity of the CFS subject pool that we study.

We have carried out a number of studies to compare this group of CFS patients with MS, depressed, and healthy controls on a variety of measures (e.g., DeLuca, Johnson, Beldowicz, & Natelson, 1995; Johnson, DeLuca, & Natelson, 1996; Johnson, DeLuca, & Natelson, in press a; Johnson, DeLuca, & Natelson, in press b; Natelson, et al., 1995). MS patients were chosen for comparison because this disease has a known organic etiology with a set of symptoms similar to those of CFS, including fatigue, depression, and cognitive dysfunction. For inclusion in our studies, patients were required to have a diagnosis of definite MS (Poser, et al., 1983) and have mild physical symptoms as determined by an expanded disability status score (EDSS) of 3.5 or less (Kurtzke, 1983). Patients with such scores are mildly affected, and their illness is difficult to identify without a careful neurological history and physical examination. We purposely chose persons with mild MS for comparison, with the expectation that our CFS patients would be far more disabled. Then, if in spite of this, the CFS and MS subjects resembled one another on our research measures, it would reinforce the idea that CFS may resemble a neurological disorder.

We chose depressive patients (DEP) as the second comparison group in order to assess the hypothesis that CFS represents a form of affective disorder. Patients chosen for the depression group had to be in good physical health and have a DSM-III-R diagnosis of depression or dysthymia, as assessed by the Quick Diagnostic Interview Schedule (Q-DIS) (Marcus, Robins, & Bucholz, 1990). Healthy control subjects were included only if they had no reported physical or psychiatric problems, and were taking no medications other than birth control pills. Exclusion criteria for all subject groups included a regular exercise regimen (in order to control for the possible role of physical inactivity in CFS symptomatology); a medical diagnosis in the five years before participation in the study or onset of illness; loss of consciousness for more than five minutes, or a history of bipolar affective disturbance, eating disorder, schizophrenia, or substance abuse as assessed by the Q-DIS. Patients with CFS and MS were obtained from the Fatigue Research and MS Centers, respectively, at UMDNJ–New Jersey Medical School. Healthy controls and DEP patients were recruited from local communities and colleges, or from local therapists, and were paid for their participation.

2. RESULTS OF RESEARCH FROM THE UMDNJ FATIGUE RESEARCH CENTER

Our research has compared the four subject groups on measures of functional status, psychiatric symptomatology, and neuropsychological impairment. In addition, other studies in our laboratory have used a variety of approaches to stratify the CFS subject pool (e.g., based on the presence or absence of psychiatric disturbance), and to compare these subgroups to one another and to healthy controls on some of the same measures. The next three sections review our CFS research on functional status, psychiatric disturbance, and neuropsychological impairment.

2.1. Functional Status

The dramatic disabling impact of CFS, as compared to other fatiguing illnesses, was clearly evident in a study which examined the functional status of the subjects (Natelson, et al., 1995). On the Illness Severity Scale, where patients rate the severity of their symptoms and the impact of their illness on their normal activities, CFS patients reported higher levels of disability than either of the other fatiguing illness groups (i.e., MS, DEP) as well as controls. Their median score was indicative of moderately severe symptoms at rest that increase with activity or exercise, leading to a 50%-70% reduction of overall activity, and the ability to work part-time at a job allowing periods of rest. Functional disability was further elaborated on the Functional Status Questionnaire (FSQ) (Jette, et al., 1986), on which CFS patients were again significantly more impaired compared to the MS, DEP, and Control groups. CFS patients reported spending more days in bed, and indicated a decreased ability to carry out basic and intermediate activities of daily living, perform work related duties, do housework, or interact socially. Despite these disabilities, CFS patients reported similar numbers of close friends as controls and MS patients, while DEP patients reported significantly fewer.

In summary, CFS patients reported significantly more functional disability than any of the other fatiguing illness groups, even DEP patients who are known to be considerably impaired functionally (Wells, et al., 1989). However, CFS subjects continued to maintain close friendships, unlike depressives.

2.2. Psychiatric Disturbance

The four groups were also compared on measures of psychiatric disturbance and mood (Natelson, et al., 1995). The Q-DIS was used to measure concurrent psychiatric disturbance at time of illness onset according to Axis I DSM-III-R criteria. CFS and MS groups did not differ in the prevalence of Axis I disorder (Comparisons were not made to DEP or control subjects since an Axis I disorder was a criterion for inclusion in the DEP group, and a criterion for exclusion in the control group). Mood was assessed with the Profile of Mood States (POMS) (McNair, Lorr, & Droppeleman, 1971). The POMS provides six subscales of mood (i.e., tension/anxiety, depression/dejection, anger/hostility, confusion, vigor, fatigue) and CFS patients were significantly different from healthy controls on each. CFS patients resembled MS patients on half of the POMS subscales, and DEP patients on the other half. In terms of tension/anxiety, depression/dejection, and anger/hostility, patients with CFS displayed an elevation similar to those with MS, but significantly below levels found among DEP subjects. In contrast, CFS patients significantly differed from the MS group and resembled the DEP group on other aspects of mood, but only on measures which are part of the case definition of CFS, i.e., increased confusion, lowered vigor, and elevated fatigue. The overwhelming fatigue experienced by CFS patients was particularly evident on the Fatigue Severity Scale (Krupp, LaRocca, Muir-Nash, & Steinberg, 1989) on which they were elevated compared to all other groups. Overall, CFS patients appeared similar on the POMS to those with MS, except on symptoms overlapping with clinical depression, on which they resembled DEP patients.

A second comparative study from our laboratory focused specifically upon depressive symptomatology among the three fatiguing illness groups (i.e., CFS, MS, DEP), as measured by the Beck Depression Inventory (BDI) (Johnson, et al., in press a). As expected, the DEP group displayed the highest average total BDI score. CFS subjects scored significantly below the DEP group and higher than the MS group on the BDI, in a range indicative of mild depression. In addition to examining total BDI score, four categories of depressive symptoms were also derived from the BDI items: mood, self-reproach, vegetative, and somatic (Huber, Freidenberg, Paulson, Shuttleworth, & Christy, 1990). No significant differences were found among the three groups on items measuring mood (e.g., sadness, discouragement) or vegetative (e.g., sleep & appetite disturbance) symptoms as a percentage of total BDI score. The CFS and MS groups displayed a higher percentage of somatic (e.g., fatigue, ability to work) symptoms than the depressed group (See Figure 1), while in comparison the depressed group exhibited the highest percentage of self-reproach (e.g., guilt, feelings of failure) symptoms (See Figure 2). These results support the contention that the type of depressive symptoms, when found in CFS patients, differ from those found in patients with clinical depression.

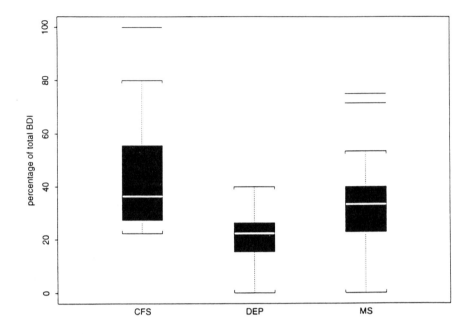

Figure 1. Box plots for somatic symptoms as a percentage of total Beck Depression Inventory score. The box depicts the interquartile range of each data set, the white horizontal bar within each box is the median, and the vertical dashed line represents the furthest data point within a range that extends 1.5 times the interquartile; this point is approximately 2.7 standard deviations beyond the mean. Points lying beyond that distance are outliers and are indicated with horizontal lines (Velleman & Hoaglin, 1981). Reprinted from Johnson, et al. (in press a), with kind permission of Elsevier Science–NL, Sara Burgerhartstraat 25, 1055 KV Amsterdam, The Netherlands.

Personality variables were more closely examined in another comparison study (Johnson, et al., in press b). DSM-III-R Axis II personality disorders and trait neuroticism were specifically examined, as measured by the PDQ-R (Hyler & Reider, 1987) and the NEO Neuroticism scale (Costa & McCrae, 1985), respectively. Neuroticism was chosen for measurement because elevations on this personality dimension have been associated with increased subjective health complaints (Costa & McCrae, 1987). The

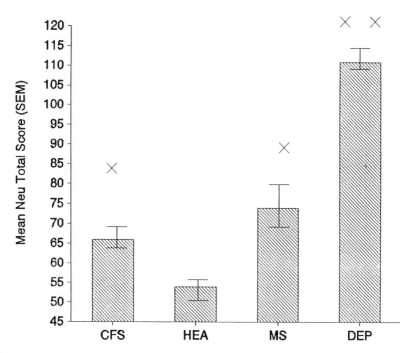

Figure 2. Box plots for self-reproach symptoms as a percentage of total Beck Depression Inventory score. Reprinted from Johnson, et al. (in press a), with kind permission of Elsevier Science–NL, Sara Burgerhartstraat 25, 1055 KV Amsterdam, The Netherlands.

high rates of such complaints among CFS sufferers suggests that neuroticism may be an important personality factor in this patient group. CFS patients were found to display an elevated level of neuroticism as compared to controls, but no higher than MS, and markedly less than depressives (See Figure 3). Thus CFS subjects exhibited levels of neuroticism typical of patients with the known organically induced fatigue brought on by MS, and not similar to the affective disorder group.

The PDQ-R, in addition to diagnosing specific DSM-III-R personality disorders, provides a total score which measures overall level of personality disturbance. As observed for the data on neuroticism, CFS subjects were found to display an elevated overall level of disturbance relative to

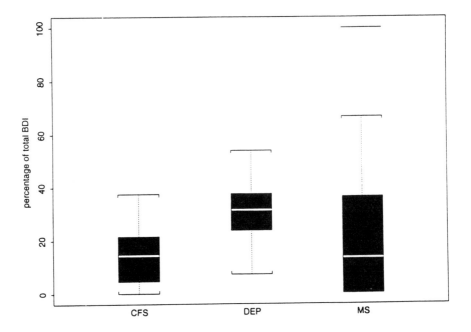

Figure 3. NEO Neuroticism Scale Total Scores (mean + or − SEM). Classification: 25–34=very low; 35–44=low; 45–54=average; 55–64=high; >=65=very high. Reprinted from Johnson, et al. (in press b) with kind permission of Elsevier Science. X = significantly higher than healthy (Fisher's PLSD, p<.05) X X = significantly higher than all three groups (Fisher's PLSD, p<.05).

controls, a level similar to that of the MS group, and significantly lower than that of depressives. The most common personality disorders in the CFS group were histrionic and borderline, in the MS group paranoid and borderline, and in the DEP group paranoid, avoidant, self-defeating, and histrionic.

In order to more closely examine the relationship of depression to personality disturbance, the CFS group was stratified into those with and those without an Axis I diagnosis of depression concurrent with illness onset, as measured by the Q-DIS. The depressed CFS group was found to score significantly higher than their non-depressed CFS counterparts on the NEO and marginally higher (p<.06) on the PDQ-R total score. Furthermore, when the non-depressed CFS subgroup was compared with healthy controls there were no significant differences on either the NEO or the PDQ-R. These results indicate that personality disturbance, when present in CFS, tends to be found specifically among a subgroup of CFS patients who are also concurrently clinically depressed. Thus, it appears that symptoms of psychiatric disturbance tend to cluster in a subgroup of CFS patients. The findings suggest the utility of classifying CFS patients on the basis of concurrent psychiatric disturbance, even within this relatively homogeneous pool of subjects chosen to have been psychiatrically intact prior to illness onset.

2.3. Neuropsychological Impairment

CFS patients commonly complain of neuropsychological disturbance. Up to 85 percent of patients report cognitive impairment, often involving the areas of concentration and memory (Komaroff, 1993). Neuropsychological functioning has been a particular focus of research in our laboratory. We have compared CFS patients with healthy controls and other fatiguing illness groups (DEP and MS) on a variety of neuropsychological tasks (DeLuca, et al., 1995). Included were measures of subjective cognitive complaints (Cognitive Problems Checklist, Metamemory Questionnaire) as well as a range of neuropsychological tasks, including higher cognitive functions (Booklet Category Test <BCT> and WAIS-R subtests of Vocabulary, Arithmetic, Similarities, & Block Design), with a particular emphasis on objective testing in the areas that CFS patients complain about most: attention and concentration (Paced Auditory Serial Attention test <PASAT>, Trails A & B, WAIS-R Digit Span), and memory (California Verbal Learning Test <CVLT>, Rey-Osterreith Complex Figure <ROCF>, and Logical Memory from the Wechsler Memory Scale–Revised <WMS-R>).

CFS patients had the greatest amount of cognitive complaints, even more so than depressives, with subjective difficulties in the areas of attention, concentration, memory, and reasoning. Objectively, however, the deficits of the CFS group were more limited. As compared to healthy controls, CFS subjects displayed a deficit in sustained selective processing of complex auditory information (PASAT total score), but no impairment on less demanding tasks of attention and concentration (WAIS-R Digit Span, Trails A & B). In addition, the CFS patients exhibited a deficit in the acquisition of verbal information during memory testing (CVLT learning trials 1–5). However, they did not display impaired recall of information once it had been learned (CVLT free and cued delayed recall as a percentage of words learned by trial 5). The overall level of cognitive impairment of the CFS patients appeared most similar to the depressed group, based upon a cognitive impairment index that summed the standard deviations of test scores below the mean performance of the healthy controls. Importantly however, in three studies we have failed to find a relationship between depression (as measured by Beck Depression Inventory) and cognitive impairment on the PASAT (DeLuca, Johnson, & Natelson, 1993; DeLuca, et al., 1995; Johnson, DeLuca, Diamond, & Natelson, in press).

In an effort to better understand the relationship between psychiatric disturbance and cognitive processing in CFS, a study was carried out in which the CFS sample was stratified by psychiatric status (DeLuca, Johnson, Ellis, & Natelson, submitted). CFS patients were categorized into two groups, those with a concurrent (post illness onset) DSM-III-R psychiatric disorder (CFS psych) and those without (CFS no-psych), as measured by the Q-DIS. Stratification of this kind is critical because of the hypothesis that CFS cognitive deficits may be secondary to psychiatric disturbance (Krupp, Sliwinski, Masur, Friedberg, & Coyle, 1994). Such a hypothesis would predict that CFS psych group would perform more poorly on cognitive tasks than their non-psychiatrically disturbed counterparts. The two groups were found to be demographically similar in terms of mean age, education, and gender distribution. The primary Axis I diagnosis in the CFS psych group was major depression (73%), while other disorders included panic disorder (26%), phobia (26%), dysthymia (13%), generalized anxiety disorder (20%), and somatoform disorder (6%). The neuropsychological tasks chosen were largely the same as those in the study above (DeLuca, et al., 1995), with measures of higher cognitive functioning, attention, concentration, and memory.

Contrary to the belief that CFS cognitive impairment is a secondary response to psychiatric disturbance, the data indicated that the CFS no-psych group was the most cognitively impaired. Compared to healthy controls, the CFS psych group displayed no differences on any of the specific tasks, while the CFS no-psych group was significantly impaired on measures of sustained information processing (PASAT, Digit Span Backwards) and acquisition and recall of verbal information (CVLT T-score and long delay free recall). In addition, the CFS no-psych subgroup was significantly more impaired than both the controls and CFS psych group on additional measures of visual (ROCF immediate and delayed recall) and verbal (CVLT short free recall) recall. It should be noted that while the CFS psych group did not differ from controls on any of the individual tests of cognition, a significant difference did emerge when tasks were examined as a whole (using MANCOVA), indicating that this group may also display subtle cognitive impairment. Nonetheless, the results argue that cognitive impairment in at least one subgroup of CFS sufferers cannot be explained by the presence of psychiatric disturbance. These results are particularly important in light of the recommendations of the NIH/CDC study group, which outlined the need to clarify the role of psychiatric disorders in CFS (Fukuda, et al., 1994).

In a second stratification study we attempted to select a subgroup of CFS patients whose illness was more likely to have directly resulted from an infectious or toxic agent (DeLuca, Johnson, & Natelson, submitted). CFS patients

were categorized into two subgroups based on characteristics regarding symptom onset: sudden versus gradual.
Sudden onset was defined as an acute viral-like illness
with a specific date of onset from which subjects did not
recover. Gradual onset was defined as a slow progression
of symptoms over a period of weeks to several months or
more. The sudden onset group was considered more likely
to be suffering from infection or toxicity. Mean age, education, and gender distribution did not differ between the
two groups. The neuropsychological tasks administered
were the same as in the CFS psych versus CFS no-psych
stratification study discussed above. Results indicated
that both subgroups were impaired overall (based on MAN-
COVA) in comparison to the healthy controls. Both displayed specific deficits with regard to sustained
information processing (PASAT) and visual (ROCF immediate) recall. However, only the sudden onset group displayed a deficit in verbal acquisition and recall (CVLT
T-score, short & long free recall) recall compared to controls.

   We have also examined the relationship between mode
of illness onset and psychiatric disturbance in an effort to
link the two stratification variables (DeLuca, et al., submitted). It was found that patients with a gradual onset of
symptoms were significantly more likely to suffer from Axis
I psychiatric disturbance than those with a sudden onset
(82% vs. 28%, respectively), with major depression the
most common diagnosis in both subgroups. Taken together, the results of the stratification studies point to the
possibility of at least two subgroups of CFS patients. One
subgroup with a gradual onset of symptoms, concurrent
psychiatric disturbance, and relatively mild cognitive impairment, and another subgroup with a more sudden onset, a lack of psychiatric disturbance, and more serious
cognitive deficits. At this point, the relationship and relative importance of psychiatric disturbance and mode of illness onset remain unclear. Further studies are being
undertaken to examine these issues. However, the finding
of distinctive CFS subgroups is consistent with recent

work based on multivariate analyses (principle components and latent class analysis) of CFS patients' subjective
complaint profiles (Hickie, et al., 1995).

3. SUMMARY AND CONCLUSIONS

Research in our laboratory has attempted to reduce CFS
sample heterogeneity in an effort to better understand the
causal pathways to this syndrome. We have been particularly interested in addressing the psychiatric/nonpsychiatric
etiological controversy. As stated earlier, three general possibilities have been raised with regard to the role of psychiatric
disturbance when it is present in CFS (David, 1991).
Chronic illness may lead to the development of psychiatric
disorder, psychiatric disturbance may account for the CFS
symptoms, or a third variable may cause both the psychiatric and CFS symptoms. While heterogeneity in the CFS
population makes it difficult to eliminate any of the alternatives, our research shows that DSM-III-R psychiatric disturbance does not account for many of the symptoms and
features of at least a subgroup of CFS patients.

Our research has examined a relatively homogeneous
sample of CFS patients for whom psychiatric disorder was
less likely to be a causal factor, since they had no history
of Axis I psychiatric disturbance before the onset of illness.
These CFS patients were compared to patients whose fatiguing illness was the result of psychiatric (DEP) or
nonpsychiatric (MS) factors. In addition, some of our studies went further to eliminate the possible role of psychiatric illness by subdividing the CFS group into those with
and without concurrent psychiatric disorders (i.e., post
CFS onset).

The severity of functional impairment in the overall
CFS group was found to be worse than all other patient
groups, even DEP. Unlike DEP patients, however, those
with CFS tended to maintain normal numbers of close
friends. The mood of CFS patients on the POMS resembled
those with MS, except for symptoms which overlap with

clinical depression, in which CFS appeared more like the DEP group. Similarly, CFS patients displayed a pattern of depressive symptoms on the BDI which were similar to MS (with an elevated proportion of somatic symptoms), and unlike the DEP group (which had the highest percentage of self-reproach items). Rates of concurrent Axis I psychiatric disturbance were similar to MS. Levels of Axis II personality disorders and trait neuroticism were also like MS, and significantly below DEP patients.

The overall psychiatric profile of CFS patients differed significantly from the DEP patients on a variety of measures. In many ways the CFS group resembled MS patients, who have an organically known basis for their fatigue. There was also an indication that psychiatric symptomology tended to cluster in particular CFS patients. A stratification of the CFS group revealed that a subgroup of CFS patients with a concurrent Axis I depressive diagnosis was also the most likely to suffer from personality disturbance. In contrast, CFS subjects without depression were similar to healthy controls on personality measures. Thus, there was evidence of heterogeneity within the CFS group, one subgroup with concurrent psychiatric symptomatology and the other without.

With regard to cognition, the overall group of CFS patients reported the broadest range of subjective complaints of any group. Objectively, however, their impairments were limited to acquisition and sustained selective processing of verbal material. While their specific pattern of impairment did not match that of either of the other fatiguing illness groups, the severity of their overall level of impairment was most similar to DEP patients. However, stratification of the CFS sample showed that CFS patients *without* concurrent Axis I psychiatric disorder were on average the most severely impaired cognitively. Compared with healthy controls, this subgroup displayed deficits in acquisition, sustained selective processing, and recall of verbal information. This subgroup was additionally impaired as compared to both controls and CFS psych patients on measures of visual and verbal memory. In another stratification study of cognition, CFS patients were categorized on the basis of characteristics regarding the onset of their illness. While the results were less dramatic, the subgroup with a sudden onset of symptoms appeared to suffer from a wider variety of cognitive deficits than did their counterparts with gradual onset. It was also found that the sudden onset group was less likely to suffer from a concurrent psychiatric disorder.

The overall pattern of results points to the existence of at least one CFS subgroup whose illness is probably not caused by psychiatric disturbance. This subgroup, with an absence of psychiatric disorder both before and concurrent with CFS onset, displayed the most neuropsychological impairment. The role of psychiatric disturbance is somewhat less clear for their CFS counterparts who had no history of psychiatric disorder, but who did exhibit a concurrent disorder. It does appear, however, that the psychiatric profile of CFS patients who do display such symptoms differs in many ways from DEP patients, and tends to resemble patients with MS, who have a known physical cause for their fatiguing illness. We are currently in the process of examining CFS subgroups with regard to viral and immunological markers.

It should be clearly noted that our results arise from a fairly specific CFS subject pool of moderate to severely ill individuals who had suffered for a limited period of time (<=4 years), and were not psychiatrically disturbed prior to illness. The findings may not generalize to broader samples of patients with vague complaints and previous psychiatric illness.

The results appear to support the strategy of reducing heterogeneity in CFS samples in order to better characterize the illness(es). Other studies have taken different approaches to addressing CFS sample heterogeneity, particularly as it pertains to psychiatric symptoms. A number of studies have attempted to examine the relationship between psychiatric symptoms and cognition in a variety of CFS samples, but this work has led to inconsistent results. For example, while several studies found no relationship between depression and cognition (e.g., Grafman, et al., 1993; Joyce, Blumenthal, & Wessely, 1996; Smith,

Behan, Bell, Millar, & Bakheit, 1993), others have (e.g., Krupp, et al., 1994; McDonald, Cope, & David, 1993; Ray, Phillips, & Weir, 1993). Heterogeneity of samples both within and across studies may help to account for this lack of consistency.

Katon and Russo (1992) took another approach to the issue of psychiatric illness and CFS. They studied fatigued patients who did not necessarily meet the case definition for CFS. They found that patients who reported more CFS symptoms were also more likely to have had a psychiatric illness prior to CFS onset. To eliminate psychiatric patients from CFS samples, they suggested reducing the number of symptoms required for a CFS diagnosis. Our work shows that the opposite approach, a tightening of inclusion criteria and an examination of homogeneous subgroups, may be a useful alternative. Stratification techniques have been specifically recommended by the CDC/NIH study group for the study of CFS (Fukuda, et al., 1994). Employing this strategy, the results of our investigations indicate that the illness of at least some CFS patients may have a nonpsychiatric, possibly viral/immunological origin. The challenge is to better characterize the distinguishing characteristics of CFS subgroups in terms of symptomology and etiology.

ACKNOWLEDGMENTS

This research was supported in part by grant AI-32247 from the National Institutes of Health, Bethesda, Md., establishing a Chronic Fatigue Syndrome Research Center at the University of Medicine and Dentistry of New Jersey–New Jersey Medical School, Newark, NJ.

REFERENCES

Costa, P. T., & McCrae, R. R. (1985). *The NEO personality inventory manual.* Odessa, FL: Psychological Assessment Resources.

Costa, P. T., & McCrae, R. R. (1987). Neuroticism, somatic complaints, and disease: Is the bark worse than the bite? *Journal of Personality, 55,* 299–316.

David, A. (1991). Postviral fatigue syndrome and psychiatry. *British Medical Bulletin, 47,* 966–988.

DeLuca, J., Johnson, S. K., & Natelson, B. H. (1993). Information processing efficiency in chronic fatigue syndrome and multiple sclerosis. *Archives of Neurology, 50,* 301–304.

DeLuca, J., Johnson, S. K., Beldowicz, D., & Natelson, B. H. (1995). Neuropsychological impairments in chronic fatigue syndrome, multiple sclerosis, and depression. *Journal of Neurology, Neurosurgery, and Psychiatry, 58,* 38–43.

DeLuca, J., Johnson, S. K., Ellis, S. P., & Natelson, B. H. (submitted). Cognitive functioning is impaired in chronic fatigue syndrome patients devoid of psychiatric disease.

DeLuca, J., Johnson, S. K., & Natelson, B. H. (submitted). Sudden versus gradual onset of chronic fatigue syndrome differentiates individuals on cognitive and psychiatric measures.

Fukuda, K., Straus, S. E., Hickie, I., Sharpe, M. C., Dobbins, J. G., Komaroff, A., et al. (1994). The chronic fatigue syndrome: A comprehensive approach to its definition and study. *Annals of Internal Medicine, 121,* 953–959.

Grafman, J., Schwartz, V., Dale, J. K., Scheffers, M., Houser, C., & Straus, S. E. (1993). Analysis of neuropsychological functioning in patients with chronic fatigue syndrome. *Journal of Neurology, Neurosurgery, & Psychiatry, 56,* 684–689.

Hickie, I., Lloyd, A., Hadzi-Pavlovic, D., Parker, G., Bird, K., & Wakefield, D. (1995). Can the chronic fatigue syndrome be defined by distinct clinical features? *Psychological Medicine, 25,* 925–935.

Holmes, G. P., Kaplan, J. E., Gantz, N. M., Komaroff, A. L., Schonberger, L. B., Straus, S. E., Jones, J. F., DuBois, R. E., Cunningham-Rundles, C., Pahwa, S., Tosato, G., Zegans, L. S., Purtilo, D. T., Brown, N., Xchooley, R. T., & Brus, I. (1988). Chronic fatigue syndrome: A working case definition. *Annals of Internal Medicine, 108,* 387–389.

Huber, S. J., Freidenberg, D. L., Paulson, G. W., Shuttleworth, E. C., & Christy, J. A. (1990). The pattern of depressive symptoms varies with progression of Parkinson's disease. *Journal of Neurology, Neurosurgery, and Psychiatry, 53,* 275–278.

Hyler, S. E., & Reider, R. O. (1987). *PDQ-R: Personality Disorders Questionnaire-Revised.* New York: New York State Psychiatric Institute.

Jette, A. M., Davies, A. R., Cleary, P. D., Calkins, D. R., Rubenstein, L. V., Fink, A., Kosecoff, J., Young, R. T., Brook, R. H., & Delbanco, T. L. (1986). The functional status questionnaire: reliability and validity when used in primary care. *Journal of General Internal Medicine, 1,* 143–149.

Johnson, S. K., DeLuca, J., Diamond, B. J.,& Natelson, B. H. (in press). Selective impairment of auditory processing in chronic fatigue syndrome: A comparison with multiple sclerosis and healthy controls. *Perceptual and Motor Skills.*

Johnson, S. K., DeLuca, J., & Natelson, B. H. (1996). Assessing somatization disorder in the chronic fatigue syndrome. *Psychosomatic Medicine, 58,* 50–57.

Johnson, S. K., DeLuca, J., & Natelson, B. H. (in press a). Depression in fatiguing illness: comparing patients with chronic fatigue syndrome, multiple sclerosis, and depression. *Journal of Affective Disorders.*

Johnson, S. K., DeLuca, J., & Natelson, B. H. (in press b). Personality dimensions in the chronic fatigue syndrome: A comparison with multiple sclerosis and depression. *Journal of Psychiatric Research.*

Joyce, E. M., Blumenthal, S., & Wessely, S. (1996). Memory, attention, and executive function in chronic fatigue syndrome. *Journal of Neurology, Neurosurgery, and Psychiatry, 60,* 495–503.

Katon, W., & Russo, J. (1992). Chronic fatigue syndrome criteria: A critique of the requirement for multiple physical complaints. *Archives of Internal Medicine, 152,* 1604–1609.

Komaroff, A. L. (1988). Chronic fatigue syndromes: Relationship to chronic viral infections. *Journal of Virological Methods, 21,* 3–10.

Komaroff, A. L. (1993). Clinical presentation of chronic fatigue syndrome. In G. R. Bock & J. Whelan (Eds.), *Chronic fatigue syndrome.* Ciba Foundation Symposium, *173,* 43–61.

Kruesi, M. J. P., Dale, J., & Straus, S. E. (1989). Psychiatric diagnosis in patients who have chronic fatigue syndrome. *Journal of Clinical Psychiatry, 20,* 53–56.

Krupp, L. B., LaRocca, N. G., Muir-Nash, J., & Steinberg, A. D. (1989). The fatigue severity scale: Application to patients with multiple sclerosis and systemic lupus erythematosus. *Archives of Neurology, 46,* 1121–1123.

Krupp, L. B., Sliwinski, M., Masur, D. M., Friedberg, F., & Coyle, P. K. (1994). Cognitive functioning and depression in patients with chronic fatigue syndrome and multiple sclerosis. *Archives of Neurology, 51,* 705–710.

Kurtz, J. F. (1983). Rating of neurologic impairment in multiple sclerosis: An expanded disability status scale (EDSS). *Neurology, 33,* 1444–1452.

Landay, A. L., Jessop, C., Lennette, E. T., & Levy, J. A. (1991). Chronic fatigue syndrome: Clinical condition associated with immune activation. *Lancet, 338,* 707–712.

Lane, T. J., Manu, P., & Matthews, D. A. (1991). Depression and somatization in the chronic fatigue syndrome. *American Journal of Medicine, 91,* 335–344.

Manu, P., Lane, T. J., & Matthews, D. A. (1992). Chronic fatigue syndromes in clinical practice. *Psychother Psychosom, 58,* 60–68.

Marcus, S., Robins, L. N., & Bucholz, K. (1990). *Quick diagnostic interview schedule 3R, version 1.* St. Louis: Washington University School of Medicine.

McDonald, E., Cope, H., & David, A. (1993). Cognitive impairment in patients with chronic fatigue: a preliminary study. *Journal of Neurology, Neurosurgery, & Psychiatry, 56,* 812–815.

McNair, D. M., Lorr, M., & Droppleman, L. F. (1971). *Profile of mood states: Manual.* San Diego: Educational and Industrial Testing Service.

Natelson, B. H., Cohen, J. M., Brassloff, I., & Lee, H. J. (1993). A controlled study of brain magnetic resonance imaging in patients with the chronic fatigue syndrome. *Journal of the Neurological Sciences, 120,* 213–217.

Natelson, B. H., Johnson, S. K., DeLuca, J., Sisto, S., Ellis, S. P., Hill, N., & Bergen, M. T. (1995). Reducing heterogeneity in chronic fatigue syndrome: A comparison with depression and multiple sclerosis. *Clinical Infectious Diseases, 21,* 1204–1210.

Patarca, R., Klimas, N. G., Lugtendorf, S., Antoni, M., & Fletcher, M. A. (1994). Dysregulated expression of tumor necrosis factor in chronic fatigue syndrome: Interrelations with cellular sources and patterns of soluble immune mediator expression. *Clinical Infectious Diseases, 18*(Suppl 1), S147–153.

Pepper, C. M., Krupp, L. B., Friedberg, F., Doscher, C., & Coyle, P. K. A comparison of neuropsychiatric characteristics in chronic fatigue syndrome, multiple sclerosis, and major depression. *Journal of Neuropsychiatry and Clinical Neuroscience, 5,* 200–205.

Ray, C., Phillips, L., & Weir, W. R. C. (1993). Quality of attention in chronic fatigue syndrome: Subjective reports of everyday attention and cognitive difficulty, and performance on tasks of focused attention. *British Journal of Clinical Psychology, 32,* 357–364.

Schluederberg, A., Straus, S. E., Peterson, P., Blumenthal, S., Komaroff, A. L., Spring, S B., Landay, A., & Buchwald, D. (1992). Chronic fatigue syndrome research: Definition and medical outcome assessment. *Annals of Internal Medicine, 117,* 325–331.

Smith, A. P., Behan, P. O., Bell, W., Millar, K., & Bakheit, M. (1993). *British Journal of Psychology, 84,* 411–423.

Strober, W. (1994). Immunological function in chronic fatigue syndrome. In S. E. Straus (Ed.) *Chronic Fatigue Syndrome* (pp. 207–237) New York: Marcell Dekker, Inc.

Velleman, P. F., & Hoaglin, D. C. (1981). *Applications, basics, and computing of exploratory data analysis.* Boston: Duxbury Press.

Wells, K. B., Stewart, A., Hays, R. D., Burnam, M. A., Rogers, W., Daniels, M., Berry, S., Greenfield, S., & Ware, J. (1989). The functional and well-being of depressed patients. Results from the Medical Outcomes Study. *Journal of the American Medical Association*, *262*, 914–919.

Wessely, S. (1994). The history of chronic fatigue syndrome. In S. E. Straus (Ed.) *Chronic Fatigue Syndrome* (pp. 3–44). New York: Marcell Dekker, Inc.

5

NONRESTORATIVE SLEEP, MUSCULOSKELETAL PAIN, FATIGUE, AND PSYCHOLOGICAL DISTRESS IN CHRONIC FATIGUE SYNDROME, FIBROMYALGIA, IRRITABLE BOWEL SYNDROME, TEMPORAL MANDIBULAR JOINT DYSFUNCTION DISORDERS (CFIT)

Harvey Moldofsky

University of Toronto Centre for Sleep And
    Chronobiology
The Toronto Hospital, Western Division
399 Bathurst Street, Toronto, Canada M5T 2S8

ABSTRACT

Nonrestorative sleep, chronic fatigue, musculoskeletal pain, and psychological distress characterize patients with the diagnostic labels of Chronic Fatigue Syndrome, Fibromyalgia, Irritable Bowel Syndrome, and Temporomandibular Joint Disorder. These labels are simplified with the acronym **CFIT**. **CFIT** disorders share the ignominy of a lack of evidence for any structural disease or specific psychiatric disorder. **CFIT** occur more often in women. **CFIT** patients share additional features that include: variable diffuse myalgia, organ and environmental hypersensitivity, psychological distress, and disturbed

Chronic Fatigue Syndrome, edited by Yehuda and Mostofsky
Plenum Press, New York, 1997

sleep physiology. A chronobiological theoretical model of **CFIT** functional pathology is described whereby there is a disturbance in the sleeping-waking brain and its interrelationship with neurotransmitter, neuroendocrine, thermal, and immune functions.

INTRODUCTION

The notion that nonrestorative sleep is inextricably linked to bodily pain, fatigue, and psychological distress has been known long before diagnostic classification of illness became fashionable. The description of this malaise condition was recorded on ancient Sumerian clay tablets, more than four thousand years ago. In the epic of Gilgamish, the hero complains, "my face was not sated with sweet sleep, I fretted myself with wakefulness, I filled my joints with misery" (McAlpine, 1987). Advances in technology have allowed us to gain new insights on the hitherto mysterious operations of the sleeping-waking brain and have helped us understand our inherent circadian behavioural and physiological rhythms. The applications of the new technologies now enable us to determine what happens to the body and mind when the rhythms of the body are perturbed and the natural restorative functions of sleep are disrupted. Such disruptions of bodily and mental functions are evidenced in patients who carry a variety of diagnostic labels that attempt to categorize such people who have no demonstrable evidence for disease. Therefore, the objectives of this chapter are to review the following:

1. how current notions of disease have not furthered our understanding of those illnesses that are characterized by chronic pain, fatigue, unrefreshing sleep and psychological distress, i.e., chronic fatigue syndrome, fibromyalgia, irritable bowel syndrome, and temporomandibular joint dysfunction;
2. how these currently fashionable diagnostic labels that are thought to explain differing ailments share essential common clinical features;

3. how current research on the perturbations of the sleeping - waking brain contribute to the understanding and management of those ailments of people whose faces are not sated with sweet sleep, and whose bodies and mind are wracked with pain, fatigue and misery.

The Failure of Current Notions of Disease to Explain Chronic Fatigue Syndrome, Fibromyalgia, Irritable Bowel Syndrome, and Temporomandibular Joint Dysfunction

Current notions of disease subscribe to the view that there is scientific evidence for an alteration in normal bodily functions. The evidence comes from systematic clinical observations and supported by laboratory demonstrations of structural and/or functional changes that can be attributed to a constellation of complaints. A common medical dilemma is how to categorize a patient who perceives unpleasant sensations but does not show any objective clinical or laboratory evidence that could be attributed to known disease. The dilemma is acceptable for those patients whose complaints can be systematically categorized by the physician as falling within the framework of psychiatry. However, even among psychiatrists the label of mental disease is problematic where there is no laboratory evidence for structural alterations of the brain or metabolic disturbance that can be linked to the symptoms. In such circumstances the notion of "disease" is replaced by one of "disorder", e.g., in mental disorder or personality disorder as described in the American Psychiatric Association's Diagnostic and Statistical Manual of Mental Disorders or DSM (1987). Difficulties arise where the complaints imply a disturbance in bodily functions as with pain, weakness, and fatigue, but nothing can be found to account for such symptoms.

Early in psychiatric history these ailments were attributed to hysteria, but during the latter half of this century hysteria fell out of favour. The term has been replaced by

Somatoform Disorder where the belief is that fundamental psychological disturbance is at the root of patients' complaints of physical ailments or incapacities where no disease can be demonstrated. In the DSM IIIR, such patients with Somatoform Disorders are subcategorized as Somatization Disorder where there is a multiplicity of complaints, Somatoform Pain Disorder where the complaint is pain, or as Neurasthenia if the attention is directed to weakness and fatigue. Previously, in DSM III the diagnostic term Psychogenic Pain Disorder implied that psychological factors could be attributed to the etiology or perpetuation of the bodily complaints. However, in the DSM IIIR description of Somatoform Pain Disorder the features were described in this paradoxical way: "In the cases there may be evidence that psychological factors are etiologically involved in the pain, ... In still other cases there may be no direct evidence of an etiologic role of psychological factors" (DSM-III-R, 1987).

What then is the role of psychological disturbance in this purported psychiatric diagnosis of mental illness? In their deliberations the authors of the newly revised DSM IV acknowledged the difficulty in requiring an etiological psychological connection to the complaints of pain (Task force on DSM IV, 1991). There were other serious problems with Somatoform Pain Disorder. It may be impossible to determine whether the severity of pain is in excess of what could be expected if there was an underlining medical condition. The medical condition that caused the pain was not as yet detectable. Even if the pain was related to a disease, the pain may respond to psychotropic drugs or psychological treatment. Therefore, the Task Force opted for a broad category, Pain Disorder within the Somatoform Disorders section of classification. The Task Force saw several advantages: it would provide the clinician with the opportunity to decide on the psychological factors that may be presumed to be responsible for the pain; it would avoid the difficulties of the differential diagnosis of pain; the impossible clinical judgment of the significance of severity of pain would be eliminated. However, by classifying the Pain

Disorder within the Somatoform category, DSM IV does not avoid the psychiatric bias that the pain is essentially rooted in a psychological construct despite the somatic focus of the complaint.

Once again the category of Somatoform Disorder is applied as an umbrella to safeguard psychiatry's lack of understanding of patients whose primary focus is fatigue. The nineteenth century term "Neurasthenia" as a descriptive label for those afflicted with such a malady was eliminated from DSM III because the term could not be easily differentiated from Somatoform, Anxiety, and Depressive Disorders as well as nonpsychiatric medical conditions. Changing fashion resulted in Neurasthenia being rarely used as a diagnosis. Despite these admonitions, the Task Force included Neurasthenia within the Somatoform Disorders. They decided to reinsert the label because Neurasthenia continued to be used in the International Classification of Disease (ICD 9 and ICD 10); they could not fit such complaints in another category of mental disorder; neurasthenia might be a convenient label to include those people with somatic, anxiety and depressive symptoms. As with Pain Disorder the Task Force acknowledged the lack of psychiatric understanding of people who are given such labels. They conferred their legitimacy to the return of the diagnosis to DSM IV because it was used in other cultures, e.g., China. They added to the confusion by claiming that it was "a frequent presentation in primary care settings, e.g., chronic fatigue syndrome." It would be better to restrict the psychiatric label of somatoform disorder to those patients who show obvious clinical evidence of mental disturbances that relate to the expression of their physical complaints, e.g., severe depression or anxiety. We should not assume that their health problems are fundamentally mental and unconscious in such patients with no clinical and laboratory evidence for disease and therefore, hidden from the enquiring physician

The patients with diffuse musculoskeletal pain, fatigue, unrefreshing sleep and psychological distress populate various specialist practices because of the belief that the symptoms reflect some, as yet, undetectable disease that is of specialized interest to the physician. The problems of diagnostic classification and lack of understanding that prevail in psychiatry, also prevail in such specialties as neurology, rheumatology, infectious disease, gastroenterology, allergy, urology, cardiology, and dentistry. These specialty groups have adopted their own diagnostic constructs that are based on their belief systems as to the physical origin of the symptoms. Depending upon the influence of the specialty and public acceptance, the diagnostic label acquires a fashionable reputation as to the presumed etiology that fits the interest of the specialty group.

The rheumatological interest grew shortly after the turn of this century out of the initial belief in an inflammation of fibrous tissue that was proposed to affect people with unexplained rheumatic ailments. In an address to the National Hospital for the Paralysed and Epileptic, Sir William Gowers, a neurologist, suggested that lumbago and similar forms of muscular rheumatism were the result of inflammation of fibrous tissue, hence the term, "Fibrositis" (Gowers, 1904). Histological evidence for inflammation in tender "fibrositis nodules" by Stockman in Edinburgh (Stockman, 1904) provided initial support and subsequent popularization of the term. Later studies did not confirm the tissue findings. The diagnosis persisted well into the 1980's as a convenient label to describe patients with rheumatic complaints for which there was no pathological evidence for disease. The term, fibrositis was acknowledged by rheumatologists to be a misnomer because no evidence for inflammation of fibrous tissue could be found. The descriptive label, "Fibromyalgia" has now replaced fibrositis. However, this label implies that the focus of interest is pain in fibrous tissue and muscles, but patients are equally distressed by their unrefreshing sleep, fatigue and psychological difficulties.

Like fibromyalgia, myalgic encephalomyelitis or chronic fatigue syndrome (CFS) has a murky and controversial historical legacy (Shorter, 1993). Both were thought to be the result of agents that caused a chronic inflammatory reaction in the body. Because such symptoms may follow infectious disease such as infectious mononucleosis, a viral etiology became the focus of concern. Initially, there was interest in the Epstein-Barr virus, but when this agent could not be identified to be specific for the complaints (Holmes, Kaplan, Gantz, Komaroff, & Schonenberger, 1988; Whelton, Salit, & Moldofsky, 1992) the idea was set aside that a specific infectious agent caused the symptoms. The term CFS came into existence as the product of the concern of a group of experts in infectious diseases. They set about to establish an initial set of working criteria to describe their fatigued patients, many of whom had no definite history of a precipitating infectious disease or any known cause for their complaints of pervasive low energy and persistent profound fatigue (Holmes, Kaplan, Gantz, Komaroff, & Schonenberger, 1988). Subsequently, these descriptive criteria were subject to a series of modifications and clarifications (Schleuderberg, Straus, Peterson, Blumenthal, Komaroff, Spring, Landay, & Buchwald, 1992; Sharpe, Archard, Banatvala, Borysiewicz, Clare, David, Edwards, Hawton, et al., 1991). These refinements resulted in the most recent consensus from an international multidisciplinary group of researchers (Fukuda, Straus, Hickie, Sharpe, Dobbins, & Komaroff, 1994). The current criteria acknowledge overlap features of CFS with fibromyalgia. Whereas pain and tenderness are the focus of concern for patients with fibromyalgia, chronic disabling fatigue is foremost for those labelled with CFS. Yet, patients from a rheumatological practice and those from an infectious disease clinic were found to share similar symptoms of chronic fatigue, myalgia, cognitive impairment, psychological distress, disturbed and unrefreshing sleep in the absence of a specific causal agent (Goldenberg, 1989).

Similarly, irritable bowel syndrome (IBS), a disorder of bowel function that is of concern to gastroenterologists, and temporomandibular joint disorder (TMD) that is of concern to dentists, share many of their nonspecific clinical features with CFS and fibromyalgia (Goldenberg, 1989;

Yunus, Masi, & Aldag, 1989; Veale, Kavanaugh, Fielding, & Fitzgerald, 1991; Triadafilopoulos, Simms, & Goldenberg, 1991; Moldofsky, & Lue 1993; Dao, Lavigne, Charbonneau, Feine, & Lund, 1994). Once more, both specialty groups of gastroenterology and dentistry have focussed their concern on the presumed organ or structure of the body that is thought to be defective in their patients. Despite efforts to identify pathology in these regions of the body, no specific structural damage has been found. Yet for convenience, the specialties prefer labels that describe functional disturbances in the bowel or jaw with labels of IBS and TMD.

The terminology continues to proliferate as the patients migrate to various medical or surgical specialties. Their variable symptoms appear to affect various regions of the body at differing and unpredictable times or are experienced as organ sensitivities, so that physiatrists have patients with diffuse "myofascial pain syndrome"; allergists have their patients with "environmental sensitivities"; urologists are concerned for their patients with an "irritable bladder"; for more than the past hundred years cardiologists describe patients with various labels including: soldier's heart, irritable heart, neurocirculatory asthenia, effort syndrome, cardiac neurosis, and if chest wall pain and tenderness are evident, Tietze's syndrome.

COMMON CLINICAL FEATURES IN CFIT DISORDERS

All these diagnostic labels share the ignominy of uncertain pathogenesis where a specific etiologic agent or localized structural pathology have not been found. Because people with these diagnoses frequent various medical, psychiatric and dental subspecialties, I have chosen to apply the acronym "**CFIT**" (**C**hronic fatigue syndrome, **F**ibromyalgia, **I**rritable bowel syndrome, **T**emporomandibular joint disorder) to describe such patients (CFIT patients), and their medical or dental specialists (CFIT specialists). In addition to the absence of clear evidence of indices of disease such as inflammatory or structural pathology, CFIT patients share a number of clinical features:

1. The symptoms of CFIT are common. A majority of patients that carry the CFIT labels are women. The prevalence of CFS is uncertain because of the varying criteria that have been employed to characterize the disorder. On the basis of a physician referral-based survey, the Centers for Disease Control in the United States claim a minimal prevalence of four to 10 cases per 100,000 adults. A majority are women in the age span of 25 to 45 years (Centers for Disease Control and Prevention, 1995).

   The newly established American College of Rheumatology criteria for fibromyalgia has resulted in community studies in various parts of the world that have used the standard criteria of widespread pain in combination with tenderness in 11 or more of 18 specific tender point sites (Wolfe, Smythe, Yunus, Bennett, Bombardier, Goldenberg, Tugwell, Campbell, et al., 1990). These studies show a prevalence of fibromyalgia in 2–4% of the population with more than 90% of adult cases occurring in women (Wolfe, 1993b). Buskila, Press, Gedalia, Klein, Neumann, Boehm, and Sukenik (1994) found a tendency for an increased prevalence in female school-age children, and showed greater tenderness to the application of a dolorimeter to tender and nontender control sites in these girls.

   Bowel dysfunctional symptoms are reported to affect between eight and 22% of the population (Drossman, Sadler, McKees, & Loveth, 1982; Sandler, Drossman, Nathan, & McKee, 1984), but 2.9% have IBS in the United States (Sandler, 1990). Women are 3.2 times more likely than men to have IBS (Sandler, 1990).

   Similarly women outnumber men in seeking

help for TMD by a ratio of 5:1. Such women are most likely to complain during the ages of 25 and 44 years, with a prevalence in that age group of 18% to 25% (Dworkin, Huggins, LeResche, VonKorff, Howard, Truelove, & Sommers, 1990).

There is no single satisfactory explanation for the greater prevalence of the symptoms of CFIT disorders to occur in females. Possible factors include gender-related biological explanations, social role influences, and the socioeconomics of health care utilization.

2. Chronic pain and localized impaired functional disturbances may become the focus of concern in a particular region or regions of the body. Over time the pain may migrate and vary in intensity or distribution in other areas of the body with accompanied generalized weakness and functional limitations. For example, patients with fibromyalgia who relate the onset of their symptoms to a motor vehicle or industrial accident often describe first experiencing posterior neck pain that is attributed to a whiplash injury, or a work-related lumbar strain. But, after an indeterminate time their localized pain and stiffness may spread from the neck or low back to inexplicably involve distal musculoskeletal areas of the body. They may become disabled from carrying out a variety of routine domestic or work-related tasks (Wolfe, Simons, Fricton, Bennett, Goldenberg, Gerwin, Hathaway, McCain, et al., 1992; Crook & Moldofsky, 1995; Goldenberg, 1995). Similarly in TMD patients, the dentist might focus his or her concern on the discomfort and functional limitations of the temporomandibular joint region. However, such patients with myofascial or regional pain often complain of musculoskeletal symptoms in other parts of the body (Fricton, 1994). Moreover, in patients with IBS their noncolonic features, particularly, backache and lethargy differentiate them from those pa-

tients with inflammatory bowel disease (Maxton, Morris, & Whorwell, 1991). While musculoskeletal pain is an acknowledged feature of CFS, the muscle and joint aches are subsumed within the general context of viewing bodily malaise as a feature of some lingering viral illness by those interested in infectious disease.

3. CFIT patients and their specialists describe bodily hypersensitivity to noxious and/or environmental stimuli. The hypersensitivity is perceived as exquisite tenderness when pressure is applied to specific anatomic regions of the surface of the body as in patients with fibromyalgia, or as intolerance to bright light, and noise. In such patients the hypersensitivities often involve seasonal climatic changes so that pain and fatigue symptoms flare during cold damp or humid weather, and relief is achieved with a dry, warm climate or applications of heat. Or, the hypersensitivity may be attributed to certain foods or noxious inhalants that trigger migraine headache or pain and motor responses from internal organs such as the bowel and bladder (Trimble, Farouk, Pryde, Douglas, & Heading, 1995; Jones & Lydeard, 1992). The sensitivities may not be confined to a particular organ or system. They may become generalized as in "multiple chemical sensitivities" where symptoms arise in the presence of low levels of exposure to those noxious agents that are thought to induce the illness. A subset of patients with CFS reported similar number of chemical sensitivities to those who claim that they had multiple chemical sensitivities (Fielder, Kippen, DeLuca, Kelly-McNeil, & Natelson, 1996). Because of the clinical similarities of fibromyalgia, CFS, and multiple chemical sensitivity, several authors suggest that these presumed separate diagnostic entities are similar conditions (Buchwald & Garrity, 1994; Kavanaugh, 1995).

4. Psychological distress is frequent and is typically construed to be evidence of an underlying psychiatric disorder. Major depressive symptoms are confounding features that are difficult to disengage from the emotional distress that results from the pain, fatigue, and poor sleep. Because of the similarity to the symptoms of depression, Hudson and Pope (1994) speculate that CFIT disorders are aspects of an Affective Spectrum Disorder. However, their theory rests on the fallacious proposition that these disorders respond to "antidepressant" medications. So-called antidepressant drugs carry a variety of biological effects that occur as the result of alterations in neurotransmitter functions. These altered neurotransmitter functions of the central and peripheral nervous system influence sleep physiology, autonomic functions, e.g., gastrointestinal motility, as well as subjective experiences including appetite, pain, energy, and mood, all of which are affected in CFIT patients. This theory leads the authors to include cataplexy as a variety of Affective Spectrum Disorder, but the neurophysiological mechanisms that result in the control of cataplexy, stem from the rapid eye movement (REM) suppressant effect of such medications and not any mood altering effects. The theory reflects a psychiatric bias for an etiological role for mood disorder as the basis for CFIT. Indeed, systematic clinical studies have not shown that depressive symptoms play a primary role in these disorders (Yunus, 1994).

There has been no easy way to differentiate between those patients whose symptoms suggest that their pain behaviour is the result of a somatoform disorder, i.e., that psychosocial factors contribute to the pain behaviour, and those whose symptoms largely reflect pathophysiological disturbances, i.e., fibromyalgia. Our studies of sleep physiology, and self ratings of pain, mood, fatigue, psychological distress, and somatic symptoms show that despite similar ratings of fatigue and pain severity in those patients with fibromyalgia, somatoform pain patients complain of more depression and overall psychological distress. However, somatoform pain patients rate themselves as having a better quality of sleep and show reduced electroencephalographic physiological arousal disturbances in their nocturnal sleep physiology (Moldofsky, Enchin, Tobin, & Lue, 1996).

5. The diffuse pain, chronic fatigue, psychological distress that afflict people with CFIT suggests that central nervous system pathophysiological mechanisms are involved in these disorders. A fundamental operation of the brain involves the sleep-wake behaviour. It is not surprising that sleep disturbances and unrefreshing sleep are common complaints of patients with CFIT. More than 90% of patients with fibromyalgia and CFS describe disturbed sleep (Goldenberg, 1989). Clinical studies show that the sleep disturbances are intimately related to the somatic symptoms and not to personality. Kolar, Harz, Roumm, Ryan, Jones, and Kirchdoerfer (1989) found that the myalgia and tender points in specific anatomic regions are related to unrefreshing sleep. Jacobsen and Danneskiold-Samsoe (1989) showed that sleep quality was associated with musculoskeletal tenderness. Therefore, the poorer the sleep, the greater the number of tender points in patients with fibromyalgia. However, the number of tender points and painful regions, and the frequency of poor sleep and fatigue were not related to psychological status (Yunus, Ahles, Aldag, & Masi, 1991). In a study of patients with IBS, 74% reported poor sleep (Goldsmith & Levin, 1993). These authors found a significant correlation between morning IBS symptoms and the quality of the prior night's sleep. Sleep disturbances, in particular, nocturnal bruxism has been thought to play an etiological role in

TMD, but no systematic sleep study has been carried out on such patients.

CHRONOBIOLOGICAL MECHANISMS INVOLVING SLEEP-WAKE PHYSIOLOGY AND THE SYMPTOMS OF CFIT

In 1975, we described an alpha (7.5–11 Hz) EEG non-rapid eye movement (NREM) sleep anomaly in patients that fulfilled our criteria for fibrositis. We proposed that the alpha EEG sleep anomaly is related to the unrefreshing sleep, diffuse myalgia, numerous localized areas of tenderness in specific anatomic areas and mood symptoms (Moldofsky, Scarisbrick, England, & Smythe, 1975). We showed that such symptoms could be experimentally produced by noise-disruption of stage 4 NREM (delta, slow wave sleep [SWS]) or deep sleep in normal sedentary people (Moldofsky & Scarisbrick, 1976). Along with the emergence of musculoskeletal pain, all the affected subjects described profound fatigue. Some subjects complained of loss of appetite, nausea, diarrhoea, and depression or irritability. The somatic symptoms declined following two nights of undisturbed sleep. Recently, Older et al confirmed that noise-induced disruption of SWS was followed by generalized aching and fatigue in healthy subjects (Older, Danninc, Battafarano, Ward, Grady, Denman, & Russell, 1994). The arousal disturbance in sleep, pain, and fatigue symptoms that we artificially induced in healthy people, and observed in patients with fibromyalgia and CFS may reflect a vigilant state during sleep with daytime symptoms of nonrestorative sleep (Anch, Lue, MacLean, & Moldofsky, 1991). This sleep physiological disturbance and the coincident perception of light unrefreshing sleep results in not only a daytime hyperalgesic state, but also many of the symptoms observed in patients with CFS, fibromyalgia, and IBS. However, the symptoms were not induced by the disruption of SWS in a group of physically-fit long distance runners at the University of Toronto (Moldofsky & Scarisbrick, 1976). This observation suggests that physical fitness plays a significant role in fibromyalgia. Subsequently, a cardiovascular fitness programme has been shown to reduce tenderness (McCain, Bell, Mai, & Halliday, 1988), and increase muscle strength (Mengshoel, Komnaes, & Forre, 1992).

In addition to our own group, a number of investigators have reported on the alpha EEG disordered sleep physiology in patients with fibromyalgia (Campbell, Clark, Tindall, Forehand, & Bennett, 1983; Molony, MacPeek, Schiffman, Frank, Neubauer, Schwartzberg, & Seibold, 1986; Ware, Russell, & Campos, 1986; Simms, Gunderman, Howard, et al., 1988; Horne & Shackell, 1991; Leventhal, Naides, & Freundlich, 1991; Anch, Lue, MacLean, & Moldofsky, 1991; Jennum, Drewes, Andreasen, & Nielsen, 1993; Branco, Atalaia, & Paiva, 1994; Drewes, Nielsen, Taagholt, Bjerregard, Svendsen, & Gade, 1995). Furthermore, some patients with fibromyalgia have fragmented sleep as a result of sleep-related periodic, involuntary, arousal disturbances that occur over the course of the night. These periodic sleep-related disturbances include: periodic involuntary movement disorder (Moldofsky, Lue, Eisen, Keystone, & Gorczynski, 1986; Hamm, Derman, & Russell, 1989), sleep-related periodic K-alpha EEG sleep (MacFarlane, Shahal, Mously, & Moldofsky, 1996), and sleep apnea, especially in men (Molony, MacPeck, Schiffman, Frank, Neubauer, Schwartzberg, & Seibold, 1986; Lario, Teran, Alonso, Alegre, Arroyo, & Veijo, 1992; May, West, Baker, & Everett, 1993). Whereas, the alpha EEG sleep may be found in noncomplaining people (Scheuler, Kubicki, Marquardt, Schola, Weiss, Henkes, & Gaeth, 1988) and is not specific for patients with fibromyalgia (Moldofsky, 1990), this sleep anomaly may be a sensitive indicator for the nonrestorative sleep and daytime symptoms (Moldofsky, 1993). In fact, patients with CFS show similar disordered sleep physiologic disturbances (Whelton, Salit, & Moldofsky, 1992; Krupp, Jendorf, Coyle, & Mendelson, 1993; Morriss, Sharpe, Sharpley, Cowen, Hawton, & Morris, 1993; MacFarlane, Shahal, Mously, &

Moldofsky, 1996). We have observed such disturbances in the EEG sleep of fibromyalgia or CFS patients who also complain of IBS and/or TMD. Disturbed sleep has been reported in patients with IBS (David, Mertz, Sytnik, Raeen, Niazi, Kodner, & Mayer, 1994) and greater amounts of REM sleep were observed in a small group of patients than controls (Kumar, Thompson, Wingate, Vesselinova-Jenkins, & Libby, 1992). As yet, no comparative sleep studies have been carried out to determine whether there are sleep physiological differences among these individual diagnostic groups of patients who attend the various medical-dental specialty clinics.

In both fibromyalgia and CFS the physiological arousal disturbances during nocturnal sleep are thought to be related to the daytime symptoms of these illnesses. I have suggested that diurnal or chronobiological variations occur in the sleep and symptoms of fibromyalgia and CFS patients. Whereas normal subjects have least pain sensitivity in the morning (Procacci, 1979), patients with fibromyalgia have increased tenderness in the morning, or no overnight improvement in pain (Moldofsky, Scarisbrick, England, & Smythe, 1975). During the course of the day, we observed that fibromyalgia patients describe their least pain and fatigue between 1000h and 1400h. On the other hand, normals report optimal functioning in the morning and early evening with a tendency to reduced alertness, cognitive functioning, and performance between 1300h and 1600h (Mitler, Carskadon, Czeisler, Dement, Dinges, & Graeber, 1988). We have examined changes in cognitive performance in patients with fibromyalgia. Such patients complained of daytime fatigue and sleepiness. They showed reduced speed, but not accuracy, on complex measures of performance throughout the day (Cote, 1995). The performance tasks were selected because they have been shown to be sensitive to sleep deprivation. The impairment in these patients is similar to the findings of cognitive dysfunction in CFS (DeLuca, Johnson, & Natelson, 1993; Smith, Behan, Bell, Millar, & Bakheit, 1993; Sandman, Barron, Nackoul, Goldstein, Fidler, 1993), and in patients with TMD (Goldberg, Mock, Ichise, Proulx, Gordon, Shandling, Tsai, & Tenenbaum, 1996). Such cognitive deficits may be the result of the disordered sleep that afflicts patients with CFIT. I have theorized that the diffuse myalgia, fatigue, and psychological distress are not only related to a disorder of the sleep-wake system, but also to circadian alterations of associated biologic systems of the body. These include: neurotransmitters (e.g., serotonin, substance P), neuroimmune (e.g., interleukin-1, natural killer cell activities), neuroendocrine (e.g., hypothalamic-pituitary-adrenal/thyroid axes), and the autonomic nervous systems of patients that have been reported to be altered in patients with fibromyalgia and CFS (Moldofsky, 1994, 1995). Future research studies should aim to assess the physiological and behavioural aspects of the chronobiology of these systems. Such knowledge may provide further insights into the etiology and management of the chronic musculoskeletal pain, fatigue, nonrestorative sleep and psychological distress that afflict CFIT patients.

REFERENCES

Anch, A. M., Lue, F. A., MacLean, A. W., & Moldofsky, H. (1991). Sleep physiology and psychological aspects of the fibrositis (fibromyalgia) syndrome. *Canadian Journal of Psychology, 45*, 178–184.

Branco, J., Atalaia, A., & Paiva, T. (1994). Sleep cycles and alpha-delta sleep in fibromyalgia syndrome. *Journal of Rheumatology, 21*, 1113–1117.

Buchwald, D., & Garrity, D. (1994). Comparison of patients with chronic fatigue syndrome, fibromyalgia, and multiple chemical sensitivities. *Archives of Internal Medicine, 154*, 2049–2053.

Buskila, D., Press, J., Gedalia, A., Klein, M., Neumann, L., Boehm, R., & Sukenik, S. (1993). Assessment of non articular tenderness and prevalence of fibromyalgia in children. *Journal of Rheumatology, 20*, 368–370.

Campbell, S. M., Clark, S., Tindall, E. A., Forehand, M. E., & Bennett, R. M. (1983). Clinical characteristics of fibrositis. I. A blinded controlled study of symptoms and tender points. *Arthritis and Rheumatism, 26*, 817–824.

Centres for Disease Control and Prevention, National Center for Infections Disease (1995). The Facts About Chronic Fatigue Syndrome. U.S. Department of Health and Human Services, Public Health Service, page 3.

Cote, K. (1995). Diurnal cognitive functioning in patients with fibromyalgia. M.Sc. Thesis, Institute of Medical Sciences, University of Toronto.

Crook, J., & Moldofsky, H. (1995). Prognostic indicators of disability after a work-related musculoskeletal injury. *Journal of Musculoskeletal Pain, 3,* 155–159.

Dao, T. T. T., Lavigne, J. P., Charbonneau, A., Feine, J .S., & Lund, J. P. (1994). Comparison of pain and quality of life in bruxers and patients with myofascial pain of the masticatory muscles. *Journal of Orofacial Pain, 8,* 350–356.

David, D., Mertz, H., Sytnik, B., Raeen, H., Niazi, N., Kodner, A., & Mayer, E. A. (1994). Sleep and duodenal motor activity in patients with severe non-ulcer dyspepsia. *Gut, 35,* 916–925.

Deluca, J., Johnson, S. K., & Natelson, B. H. (1993). Information processing efficiency in chronic fatigue syndrome and multiple sclerosis. *Archives of Neurology, 50,* 301–304.

Diagnostic and Statistical Manual of Mental Disorders, 3rd-revised (DSM-III-R) (1987). American Psychiatric Association, Washington, D.C., p. 265.

Drewes, A. M., Nielsen, K. D., Taagholt, S. J., Bjerregard, K., Svendsen, L., & Gade, J. (1995). Sleep intensity in fibromyalgia: focus on the microstructure of the sleep process. *British Journal of Rheumatology, 34,* 629–635.

Drossman, D. A., Saddler, R. S., McKees, D. C., & Loveth. A. (1982). Bowel patterns among subjects not seeking health care: Use of a questionnaire to identify a population with bowel dysfunction. *Gastroenterology, 83,* 529–534.

Dworkin, S.F., Huggins, H.K., LeResche, L., VonKorff, M., Howard, J., Truelove, E., & Sommers, E. (1990). Epidemiology of signs and symptoms in temporomandibular disorders: clinical signs in cases and controls. *Journal of the American Dental Association, 120,* 273–281.

Fielder, N., Kippen, H. M., DeLuca, J., Kelly-McNeil, K., & Natelson, B., (1996). A controlled comparison of multiple chemical sensitivities and chronic fatigue syndrome. *Psychosomatic Medicine, 58,* 38–49.

Fricton, J. R. (1994). Myofascial pain. *Bailliére's Clinical Rheumatology, 8,* 857–880.

Fukuda, K., Strauss, S. E., Hickie, I., Sharpe, M. C., Dobbins, J. G., & Komaroff, A. (1994). The chronic fatigue syndrome: a comprehensive approach to its definition and study. International Chronic Fatigue Syndrome Study Group. *Annals of Internal of Medicine, 121,* 953–959.

Goldberg, M.B., Mock, D., Ichise, M., Proulx, G., Gordon, A., Shandling, M., Tsai, S., & Tenenbaum, H.C. (1996) Neuropsychological deficits and clinical features of posttraumatic temporomandibular disorders. Journal of Orofacial Pain (in press).

Goldenberg, D. L. (1989). Fibromyalgia and its relation to chronic fatigue syndrome, viral illness and immune abnormalities. *Journal of Rheumatology, 16(Suppl. 19)*, 91–93.

Goldenberg, D. L. (1995). Overlap of fibromyalgia, myofascial pain, and chronic fatigue syndrome. *Journal of Musculoskeletal Pain, 3*, 87–91.

Goldsmith, G., & Levin, J. S. (1993). Effect of sleep quality on the symptoms of irritable bowel syndrome. *Digestive Diseases and Sciences, 38*, 1809–1814.

Gowers, W.R. (1904). Lumbago: Its lesson and analogues. *British Medical Journal, 1*, 117–121.

Hamm, C., Derman, S., & Russell, I. J. (1989). Sleep parameters in fibrositis/ fibromyalgia syndrome. *Arthritis and Rheumatism, 32*, S70.

Holmes, G. P., Kaplan, J. E., Gantz, N. M., Komaroff, A. L., & Schonenberger, L. B., Straus, S.E., Jones, J.F., Dubois, R.E., Cunningham-Rundles, C., Pahwa, S., Tosato, G., Zegans, L.S., Purtilo, D.T., Brown, N., Schooley, R.T., Brus, I. (1988). Chronic Fatigue Syndrome: A working case definition. *Annals of Internal Medicine, 108*, 387–389.

Horne, J. A., & Shackell, B. S. (1991). Alpha-like activity in nonREM sleep and the fibromyalgia (fibrositis) syndrome. *Electroencephalography & Clinical Neurophysiology, 79*, 271–276.

Hudson, J. I., & Pope, H. G. (1994). The concept of affective spectrum disorder: relationship to fibromyalgia and other syndromes of chronic fatigue and chronic muscle pain. *Baillière's Clinical Rheumatology, 8*, 839–856.

Jacobsen, S., & Danneskiold-Samsoe, B. (1989). Interrelations between clinical parameters and muscle function in patients with primary fibromyalgia. *Clinics in Experimental Rheumatology, 7*, 493–498.

Jennum, P., Drewes, A. M., Andreasen, A., & Nielsen, K.D. (1993). Sleep and other symptoms in primary fibromyalgia and in healthy controls. *Journal of Rheumatology, 20*, 1756–1759.

Jones, R., & Lydeard, S. (1992). Dyspepsia in the comunity: a follow-up study. *British Journal of Clinical Practice, 46(2)*, 95–97.

Kavanaugh, A. F. (1995). Fibromyalgia or multi-organ dysesthesia. *Arthritis and Rheumatism, 37*, 180–181.

Kolar, E., Harz, A., Roumm, A., Ryan, L., Jones, R., & Kirchdoerfer, E. (1989). Factors associated with severity of symptoms in patients with chronic unexplained muscular aching. *Annals of the Rheumatic Diseases, 48*, 317–321.

Krupp, L. B., Jendorf, L., Coyle, P.K, & Mendelson, W.B. (1993). Sleep disturbances in chronic fatigue syndrome. *Journal of Psychosomatic Research, 37*, 325–332.

Kumar, D., Thompson, P. D., Wingate, D.C., Vesselinova-Jenkins, C., & Libby, G. (1992). Abnormal REM sleep in the irritable bowel syndrome. *Gastroenterology, 103*, 12–17.

Lario, B. A., Teran, J., Alonso, J. L., Alegre, J., Arroyo, I., & Veijo, J.L. (1992). Lack of association between fibromyalgia and sleep apnoea syndrome. *Annals of the Rheumatic Diseases, 51*, 108–111.

Leventhal, L. J., Naides, S. J., & Freundlich, B. (1991). Fibromyalgia and parvovirus infection. *Arthritis and Rheumatism, 34*, 1319–1324.

MacFarlane, J.G., Shahal, B., Mously, C., & Moldofsky, H. (1996). Periodic K-alpha sleep EEG activity and periodic leg movements during sleep: comparisons of clinical features and sleep parameters. *Sleep*, (in press)

Maimonides, M. (1177). *Mishneh Torah. The Book of Knowledge.*M. Hyamson (Ed. & Translater), pp. 50–52. Boys Town Jerusalem Publishers, 1962.

Maxton, D.G., Morris, J., & Whorwell, P.J. (1991). More accurate diagnosis of irritable bowel syndrome by the use of "Non-colonic" symptomatology. *Gut, 32*, 784–786.

May, K. P., West, S. G., Baker, M.R., & Everett, D.W. (1993). Sleep apnea in male patients with fibromyalgia syndrome. *American Journal of Medicine, 94*, 505–508.

McAlpine, T.H. (1987). *Sleep, Divine and Human in the Old Testament.* Academic Press, Sheffield, pp. 120.

McCain, G. A., Bell, D.A., Mai, F.M., & Halliday, P.D. (1988). A controlled study of the effects of a supervised cardiovascular fitness training program on the manifestations of primary fibromyalgia. *Arthritis and Rheumatism, 31*, 1135–1141.

Mengshoel, A. M., Komnaes, H. B., & Forre, O. (1992). The effects of 20 weeks of physical fitness training in female patients with fibromyalgia. *Clinics in Experimental Rheumatology, 10*, 345–349.

Mitler, M. M., Carskadon, M. A., Czeisler, C. A., Dement, W. C., Dinges, D. F., & Graeber, R.C. (1988). Catastrophes, sleep, and public policy: *Consensus Report. Sleep, 11*, 100–109.

Moldofsky, H. (1990). The contribution of sleep-wake physiology to fibromyalgia. In *Advances in Pain Research and Therapy.* pp. 227–240. J. R. Fricton & A. Awad (Eds.) Vol. 17, Raven Press, Ltd., New York.

Moldofsky, H. (1993). Sleep and musculoskeletal pain. In *Progress in Fibromyalgia and Myofascial Pain.* pp. 137–148. H. Vaeroy, & H. Merskey (Eds.) Elsevier Science Publishers, Amsterdam.

Moldofsky, H. (1994). Central nervous system and peripheral immune functions and the sleep-wake system. *Journal of Psychiatry and Neuroscience, 19(5),* 368–374.

Moldofsky, H. (1995). Sleep, neuroimmune and neuroendocrine functions in fibromyalgia and chronic fatigue syndrome. *Advances in Neuroimmunology, 5,* 39–56.

Moldofsky, H., Enchin, A., Tobin, L., & Lue, F.A. (1996) Sleep and symptoms in patients with somatoform disorder vs. fibromyalgia. *Sleep Research, 27,* 168.

Moldofsky, H., & Lue, F.A. (1993). Disordered sleep, pain, fatigue, and gastrointestinal symptoms in fibromyalgia, chronic fatigue and irritable bowel syndromes. In *Basic and Clinical Aspects of Chronic Abdominal Pain.* pp. 249–255. Chapt 19. E. A. Mayer, & H. E. Raybould (Eds.) Elsevier Science Publishers, Amsterdam.

Moldofsky, H., Lue, F. A., Eisen, J., Keystone, E., & Gorczynski, R.M. (1986). The relationship of interleukin-1 and immune functions to sleep in humans. *Psychosomatic Medicine, 15,* 1701–1704.

Moldofsky, H., Scarisbrick, P., England, R., & Smythe, H.A. (1975). Musculoskeletal symptoms and NonREM sleep disturbance in patients with "fibrositis syndrome" and healthy subjects. *Psychosomatic Medicine, 34,* 341–351.

Moldofsky, H., & Scarisbrick, P. (1976). Induction of neurasthenic musculoskeletal pain syndrome by selective sleep stage deprivation. *Psychosomatic Medicine, 38,* 35–44.

Molony, R. R., MacPeck, D. M., Schiffman, P.L., Frank, M., Neubauer, J.A., Schwartzberg, M., & Seibold, J.R. (1986). Sleep, sleep apnea and the fibromyalgia syndrome. *Journal of Rheumatology, 13,* 797–800.

Morriss, R., Sharpe, M., Sharpley, A.L., Cowen, P.J., Hawton, K., & Morris, J. (1993). Abnormalities of sleep in patients with the chronic fatigue syndrome. *BMJ, 306,* 1161–1163.

Older, S. A., Danninc, C. L., Battafarano, D. F., Ward, J. A., Grady, E. P., Denman, S., & Russell, I. J. (1994). Delta wave suppression and fibromyalgia symptoms in healthy subjects: A preliminary appraisal of the Moldofsky hypothesis. *Arthritis and Rheumtism, 37(Suppl.),* 349.

Procacci, P. (1979). Methods for the study of pain threshold in man. In *Advances in Pain Research and Therapy.* pp. 781–790. J. J. Bonica et al. (Eds.), Vol. 3, Raven Press, New York.

Sandler, R. S., Drossman, D. A., Nathan, H. P., & McKee, D.C. (1984). Symptom complaints and health care seeking behavior in subjects with bowel dysfunction. *Gastroenterology, 87,* 314–318.

Sandler, R.S. (1990). Epidemiology of irritable bowel syndrome in the United States. *Gatroenterology, 99,* 409–415.

Sandman, C. A., Barron, J. L., Nackoul, K., Goldstein, J., & Fidler, F. (1993). Memory deficits associated with chronic fatigue immune dysfunction syndrome. *Biological Psychiatry, 33,* 618–623.

Scheuler, W., Kubicki, S., Marquardt, J., Scholz, G., Weib, K.H., Henkes, H., & Gaeth, L. (1988). The alpha sleep pattern - quantitative analysis and functional aspects. pp. 284–286. In *Sleep '86.* W. P. Koella, F. Obál, H. Schulz, & Visser, P. (Eds.) Gustav Fisher Verlag, Stuttgart.

Schleuderberg, A., Straus, S. E., Peterson, P., Blumenthal, S., Komaroff, A. L., Spring, S.B., Landay, A., & Buchwald, D. (1992). NIH Conference. Chronic Fatigue Syndrome Research. Definition and medical outcome assessment. *Annals of Internal Medicine, 117,* 325–331.

Sharpe, M. C., Archard, L. C., Banatvala, J. E., Borysiewicz, L. K., Clare, A. W., David, A., Edwards, R. H. T., Hawton, K. E. H., Lambert, H. P., Lane, R. J. M., McDonald, E. M., Mowbray, J. F., Pearson, D. J., Peto, T. E. A., Preedy, V. R., Smith, A. P., Smith, D. G., Taylor, D. J., Tyrrell, D. A. J., Wessely, S., White, P. D. (1991). Chronic fatigue syndrome: guidelines for research. *Journal of the Royal Society of Medicine, 84,* 118–121.

Shorter, E. (1993). Chronic fatigue in historical perspective. In *Chronic Fatigue Syndrome.* pp. 6–22. G. R. Bock, & J. Whelan (Eds.). Ciba Foundation Symposium 173. J. Wiley and Sons, Chichester.

Sims, R. W., Gunderman, J., Howard, F., et al., (1988). Comparison of sleep in osteoarthritic patients and age and sex matched healthy controls. *Annals of the Rheumatic Diseases, 47,* 40–42.

Smith, A. P., Behan, P. O., Bell, W., Millar, K., & Bakheit, M. (1993). Behavioural problems associated with chronic fatigue syndrome. *British Journal of Psychology, 84,* 411–423.

Stockman, R. (1904). The causes, pathology and treatment of chronic rheumatism. *Edinburgh Medical Journal, 15,* 107–116.

Task Force on DSM IV, American Psychiatric Association (1991). *DSM-IV Options Book: Work in Progress (9/1/1991) I,* 9-I:11.

Triadafilopoulos, G., Simms, R. W., Goldenberg, D.L. (1991). Bowel dysfunction in fibromyalgia. *Digestive Diseases and Sciences, 36,* 59–64.

Trimble, K.C., Farouk, R., Pryde, A., Douglas, S., Heading, R.C. (1995). Heightened visceral sensation in functional gastrointestinal disease is not site-specific. Evidence for a generalized disorder of gut sensitivity. *Digestive Diseases & Sciences, 40(8),* 1607–1613.

Veale, D., Kavanaugh, J. F., Fielding, J. F., & Fitzgerald, O. (1991). Primary fibromyalgia and irritable bowel syndrome: different expressions of a common pathogenetic process. *British Journal of Rheumatology, 30,* 220–222.

Ware, J.C., Russell, J., & Campos, E. (1986). Alpha intrusions into the sleep of depressed and fibromyalgia syndrome (fibrositis) patients. *Sleep Research, 15*, 210.

Whelton, C. L., Salit, I., & Moldofsky, H. (1992). Sleep, Epstein-Barr virus infection, musculoskeletal pain, and depressive symptoms in chronic fatigue syndrome. *Journal of Rheumatology, 19*, 939–943.

Wolfe, F. (1993a). Fibromyalgia: On diagnosis and certainty. *Journal of Musculoskeletal Pain, 1*, 17–35.

Wolfe, F. (1993b). The epidemiology of fibromyalgia. *Journal of Musculoskeletal Pain, 1(3/4)*, 137–148.

Wolfe, F., Simons, D. G., Fricton, J., Bennett, R. M., Goldenberg, D. L. Gerwin, R., Hathaway, D., McCain, G. A., Russell, I. J., Saunders, H. O., & Skootsky, S.A. (1992). The fibromyalgia and myofascial pain syndromes: a preliminary study of tender points and trigger points in patients with fibromyalgia, myofascial pain syndrome, and no disease. *Journal of Rheumatology, 19*, 944–951.

Wolfe, F., Smythe, H. A., Yunus, M. B., Bennett, R. M., Bennett, R. M., Bombardier, C., Goldenberg, D. L., Tugwell, P., Campbell, S. M., Abeles, M., Clark, P., Fam, A. G., Farberg, S. J., Fiechtner, J. J., Franklin, C. M., Gatter, R. A., Hamaty, D., Lessard, J., Lichtbroun, A.S., Masi, A.T., McCain, G. A., Reynolds, W. J., Romano, T. J., Russell, I. J., & Sheon, R.P. (1990). The American College of Rheumatology 1990 criteria for the classification of fibromyalgia. Report of the Multicenter Criteria Committee. *Arthritis and Rheumatism, 33*, 160–172.

Yunus, M. B. (1994). Psychological aspects of fibromyalgia syndrome: a component of the dysfunctional spectrum syndrome. *Baillière's Clinical Rheumatology, 8*, 811–837.

Yunus, M. B., Ahles, T. A., Aldag, J. C., & Masi, A.T. (1991). The relationship of the clinical features with psychological status in primary fibromyalgia. *Arthritis and Rheumatism, 34*, 15–21.

Yunus, M. B., Masi, A. T., Aldag, J. C. (1989). A controlled study of primary fibromyalgia syndrome: clinical features and association with other functional syndromes. *Journal of Rheumatology, 16(Suppl 19)*, 62–71.

6

ARGUMENTS FOR A ROLE OF ABNORMAL IONOPHORE FUNCTION IN CHRONIC FATIGUE SYNDROME*

Abhijit Chaudhuri, Walter S. Watson, and
Peter O. Behan[†]

University Department of Neurology and
   Nuclear Medicine Department
Institute of Neurological Sciences
Southern General Hospital
1345 Govan Road, Glasgow G51 4TF
Tel: 0141 201 2502; Fax: 0141 201 2515
E-mail: oss1v@clinmed.gla.ac.uk

INTRODUCTION

Chronic fatigue syndrome (CFS) is a disorder that is now receiving world-wide attention from the scientific and medical communities. The precise incidence is unknown, but it has been estimated to have a prevalence of approximately one per thousand (The facts about chronic fatigue syndrome. Coordinating Committee. US Department of Health and Human Services. CDC/NCID, September 28,

* Supported by the Barclay Research Trust at Glasgow University.
† All correspondence should be sent to Peter O Behan.

Chronic Fatigue Syndrome, edited by Yehuda and Mostofsky
Plenum Press, New York, 1997

1993). It affects individuals, women more than men at the most productive time in their lives. Until now, the syndrome has been poorly defined. Recently an attempt has been made to give a comprehensive definition that can be used in studies and research but essentially this definition, which is far from perfect, is one of exclusion (Fukuda et al, 1994). The authors "support changing the name when more is known about the underlying pathophysiological process" (Fukuda et al, 1994). The patients reported in our studies all fulfilled this recent CDC criteria and also the other definitions that have also been proposed (Majeed et al, 1995, Sharpe, 1991). All of our cases were admitted as in-patients and had an exhaustive, comprehensive study to rule out all other causes of fatigue. They had several other features which should be stressed, namely all had an abrupt or acute onset, the illness was fluctuating and made worse by exercise, and all had an influenzal-like infectious episode that precipitated the onset of the illness. A number of these patients in addition had been chronically exposed to organophosphates (Behan et al 1994, Behan, 1996).

SYNDROME X & CFS

Myocarditis, with or without Bornholm-type was a common symptom in an analysis of 1,000 patients of CFS who were seen in Glasgow over the past 20 years (Behan et al, 1991). Indeed, several of our patients who initially experienced a severe chest pain have been referred to us by cardiologists and their illness was considered to be a form of angina pectoris or atypical non-cardiac chest pain. Various aetiologies of non-cardiac chest pain have been proposed from time to time, including oesophageal reflux and spasm, chest wall pain, microvascular coronary artery disease and even anxiety and hyperventilation (Klimes et al, 1990). We were struck initially by the often occurring association of patients who develop CFS with acute chest pain resembling a coronary thrombosis (Behan et al, 1988, Behan et al, 1991). All of these patients ended up in medical units and had had extensive cardiological investigations, including ECG's, isoenzyme determinations and coronary angiograms. These investigations were essentially normal but, on subsequent clinical follow-up with this type of presentation, variously termed syndrome X (Sylven, 1993, Waldenstrom et al, 1992), all these patients had a clinical course that was indistinguishable from patients who presented with an upper respiratory tract or a gastro-intestinal tract infection and went on to develop CFS. Indeed the clinical similarity was compelling since there was an increase in incidence of females and most patients developed other symptoms associated with CFS, i.e. myalgia, dysequilibrium, irritable bowel syndrome, poor concentration, sleep and neurobehavioural symptoms. Most patients with syndrome X are considered to have a non-cardiac cause of chest pain and when other conditions such as thoracic root pain, oesophageal dysmotility are excluded, then one is left with a syndrome that is identical to CFS with the exception of chest pain being the initiating symptom (Sylven, 1993, Waldenstrom et al, 1992). There are two forms of syndrome X—one with insulin resistance, hypertriglyceridaemia and obesity and the other with pure angina but without any other features other than those outlined. Our cases had no lipid or insulin abnormalities.

A significant number of cases of syndrome X therefore, strongly resemble CFS clinically. There is further data to complete this analogy since nuclear magnetic resonance spectroscopy studies of skeletal muscle in patients with syndrome X show abnormalities that are identical to those found in patients with CFS (Soussi et al, 1993). In CFS abnormal lactate production has been found after exercise (Riley et al, 1990, Lane et al, 1995). Similarly, abnormal lactate is found in patients with syndrome X (Soussi et al, 1993, Boudoulas et al 1974). Following their extensive research in this condition, Waldenström and his group have suggested that there are abnormal ionophores in the skeletal muscle and cardiac cells of patients with syndrome X (Sylven, 1993). These ionophores are capable of altering the net transport of ions across the cell membrane thus requiring the cell to upregulate its ATPase activity in order to maintain the transmembrane ionic equilibrium. Eventually, this leads to a change of the adenine nucleotide pool inside the cell. They expressed this abnormality by using the energy charge = $(ATP + 0.5ADP) / (ATP + ADP + AMP)$. This ratio was very stable when measured from most normal tissues biopsied and its value was constant at 0.9 but fell to 0.48 and 0.70 in myocardiac and skeletal muscle respectively in patients with syndrome X and abnormal thallium cardiac scans (Waldenström et al, 1993). In a series of fascinating experiments, Waldenström and colleagues showed that similar changes in energy charge to those noted in syndrome X, resulted when ionophores were introduced into suspended human erythrocytes (Engstrom et al, 1993) and also into an isolated rat heart model (Martinussen et al, 1993). Additionally, similar findings were obtained in mouse myocardium after experimental infection with Coxsackie B3 virus (Waldenström et al, 1993). All the findings suggested low intracellular ATP levels consequent to an upregulated ATPase activity. We, in examining muscle biopsies of patients with chronic fatigue syndrome, showed an increase in calcium ATPase activity in skeletal muscles (Gow et al, 1994) . These data strengthen the relationship between CFS & syndrome X and suggest that an increased energy expenditure, for whatever reason, with a consequent reduction of intra- cellular ATP and an increase in ATPase activity could account for the abnormalities found in these two conditions.

THALLIUM CARDIAC SCANS IN CFS

Waldenström and colleagues also performed cardiac thallium-201 SPECT scans on a series of syndrome X patients (SPECT= single photon computed tomography) and detected abnormalities in a significant portion (Waldenström et al, 1992). Cardiac thallium-201 SPECT scanning involves the intravenous injection of radioactive thallium-

201 which is rapidly accumulated intra-cellularly in a similar fashion to potassium (potassium, the main intra-cellular cation, would be the preferred tracer but there is no readily available radioactive form). The technique is normally used to identify areas of the myocardium which are underperfused due to major coronary artery disease (CAD) (DePasquale et al, 1988). The sections of underperfused myocardium receive less thallium-201 via the relatively reduced bloodflow through stenosed arteries are identified as areas of reduced thallium-201 uptake when the left ventricle is imaged using a gamma camera.

The abnormalities seen in syndrome X with this technique cannot be due to major coronary artery stenosis, because the patients have angiographically normal major coronary arteries. Possible explanations are high microvascular resistance resulting in low bloodflow or a change in the metabolism at the cellular level resulting in low thallium uptake by the myocardial cells. The uptake of thallium tracer has been shown in the canine heart to be related to ATPase activity and as the adenine nucleotide concentration pattern in the syndrome X patients was similar to that found in the ionophore studies and different from that found in reversible ischaemia, Waldenström proposed that the defects seen in the uptake of thallium-201 in the left ventricle of his patients could be due to a change in cell metabolism resulting from abnormal ion leakage from the cells involved rather than microvascular ischaemia (Waldenström et al, 1993).

There has been anecdotal evidence that some of our patients with CFS who presented to cardiologists with chest pain have abnormal thallium-201 SPECT scans and this, together with the symptoms overlap between syndrome X and CFS, prompted us to carry out cardiac thallium -201 SPECT scans on a small group of CFS patients. The group consisted of 8 males and 2 females, aged from 23–57 years all with CFS diagnosed by one of us (POB). Each subject underwent a cardiac thallium-201 SPECT scan (DePasquale et al, 1988). None of the patients had a recent coronary arteriogram although one patient had had a normal investigation several years before. Image analysis revealed moderate defects in the left ventricles of 7 of the 10 patients. This was shown to be significantly different from the expected incidence of abnormal results for a population of adults with the "normal" incidence of CAD, i.e. 4% (Diamond et al, 1979).

Therefore, here again we have similar results in CFS and syndrome X suggesting that the ion leakage hypothesis proposed to explain syndrome X may also have a role to play in the pathogenesis of CFS.

RESTING ENERGY EXPENDITURE & CFS

Given the possibility of an abnormal ion permeability-driven abnormality of cell energy expenditure, we have recently begun to examine the resting energy expenditure (REE) in patients with CFS. It is perhaps not fully appreciated that approximately 70% of the total energy expenditure by an individual is utilised to maintain the intracellular milieu, e.g. ion gradients, while only 30% is used for physical activity (Leibel et al, 1995). Therefore, any significant increase in REE without a compensatory increase in energy intake, i.e. food, would reduce the energy available for physical activity and could, therefore, result in a feeling of fatigue.

In a preliminary study, REE was measured by indirect calorimetry in 10 female subjects with CFS and in 6 healthy female controls. Because fat is relative inert in terms of energy expenditure, REE is usually related to lean body mass (LBM) (Nelson et al, 1992). LBM was estimated for all subjects by total body potassium, estimated by whole body counting of the naturally occurring potassium radioisotope, K-40 (Watson, 1987), and total body water obtained from bio-electrical impedance measurements (Hannan et al, 1995). When REE for the controls was stepwise-regressed against height, weight, age, TBK and TBW, only TBK and age were selected as significant regressors. This allowed REE to be predicted in terms of these variables only. When the resulting regression equation was used to predict the REE value for the CFS group, 7 out of 10 subjects had measured REE values significantly higher than those predicted. Additionally, the TBK results for the CFS patients were significantly lower than those for controls ($p<0.05$) as previously noted (Burnet et al, 1996). While these findings are provisional, the increased resting energy expenditure and the lower body potassium found in CFS patients fit with the hypothesis of abnormal ionophore formation causing increased efflux of cell potassium. The elegance of these measurements, i.e. REE and TBK was that neither required the subject to expend any physical energy and once patients were in the resting, non-sleep state, their metabolism could be measured effectively and compared against age, weight and condition matched sedentary controls

Additional evidence is now accruing that patients with CFS might have a reduced TBK (Burnet et at, 1996). TBK could be low because either intracellular potassium is reduced as a result of an abnormal permeability of cell membrane, or there is a loss of potassium-containing tissue, e.g. due to wasting of skeletal muscles. Although patients of CFS could be deconditioned, there is seldom, if ever, any wasting of the muscles and the abnormality of TBK would probably be a result of an abnormality of membrane permeability consequent to abnormal ionophores. These fit well with the other metabolic abnormalities of CFS patients such as an impaired water metabolism (Bakheit et al, 1993), the association of fatigue with idiopathic oedema (Majeed et al, 1995) and the physiological abnormalities on table tilting experiments (Bou-Holaigah et al, 1995).

DISCUSSION

Whatever may be the initiating event or the triggering factor, it is plausible that the eventual defect in CFS lies at the cellular level in view of the widespread symptomatology so commonly found in this condition. Two ways that a cell can continue to have abnormal function after a viral infection or exposure to toxin are:-

1. an abnormality of a key enzyme or a membrane protein due to a mutation at the level of the genetic machinery of the cell
2. an immune abnormality that persists and can be exacerbated from time to time (an anamnestic reaction).

There is compelling data at the moment to show that a number of different noxae can precipitate chronic fatigue syndrome. These include viruses (Behan et al, 1988), other infections (Adams, 1980), exposure to organophosphates (Behan et al, 1994, Behan, 1996) and incapacitating stress (Friedberg, 1995) . It may also occur as a result of exposure to heavy metals and other toxins (Pearn, 1995). One of the best characterised fatigue syndromes is that occurring after ciquatera fish poisoning (Pearn, 1995). Ciquatera fish poisoning is a common form of fish poisoning in the United States (Calvert et al, 1987) and in Australia (Gillespie et al, 1986) caused by the ingestion of fish contaminated by the dinoflagellate organism gambierdiscus toxicus (Pearn, 1995). This organism elaborates a number of toxins which act to open the voltage gated sodium channels in the cell membrane of both nerve and muscle (Bidard et al, 1984). Indeed, histopathological studies from affected individuals have shown oedema at the axonal Schwann's cell cytoplasm (Allsop et al, 1986). Here therefore is one example of a chronic fatigue syndrome secondary to ion channel abnormalities. Abnormal ion channels, i.e. ionophores, are created after exposure to viruses (Carrasco et al, 1993), toxins, heavy metals, and a number of noxae (Gow et al, 1994, Kagan et al, 1992). The finding that tumour necrosis factor α may create new ionophores and that cytokines are involved in CFS may be relevant (Kagan et al, 1992). We observed in our experiments that patients with CFS share identical abnormalities clinically with syndrome X patients and have abnormal thallium scans. These patients also have an abnormally higher level of resting energy expenditure. When interpreted in the light of the suggestion put forward by Waldenström and his colleagues in syndrome X, it is possible that patients with CFS have identical abnormalities and that the increase in resting energy expenditure is due to an overactive membrane ATPase, attempting to maintain normal membrane traffic and electrochemical gradient. Our future experiments and trials are designed to test this hypothesis and to look for the presence of any immune-mediated damage to any of the membrane ion channels. The sodium channel could be a likely candidate since it has already been shown that this channel could be held in a chronically open state following ciguatera fish poisoning (DiNubile et al, 1995). Alternatively, voltage-gated potassium channel could also be the primary target. As compared to the sodium channel, potassium channels are more widespread and the potassium channel associated serotonin could play a key factor in the mood changes and emotional abnormality that characterises CFS.

In this chapter, we propose that ion channels, e.g. potassium, sodium or even calcium channels are affected in patients with CFS following exposure to viruses and organophosphates. This allows us not only to put forward a hypothesis but also to explain the observed abnormalities seen in patients with this disorder. At the moment, it is premature to speculate regarding any definite lesion of the membrane ion channels but it may not be in the too distant future when CFS would be considered as an example of channelopathy like many other neurological diseases.

REFERENCES

ADAMS RD. (1980) Lassitude and asthenia. In: Principles of Internal Medicine, Ninth Edition, Section 3, Alterations in nervous function, pp74–77. Isselbacher, Adams, Braunwald, Petersdorf & Wilson (eds). McGraw-Hill Book Company, New York.

ALLSOP JL, MARINI L, LEBRIS H. (1986) Neurological symptoms and signs of ciguatera. Three cases with neurophysiological study and one biopsy. Reviews in Neurology (Paris). 142: 590–597.

BAKHEIT AMO, BEHAN PO, WATSON WS. MORTON JJ (1993). Abnormal arginine-vasopressin secretion and water metabolism in patients with postviral fatigue syndrome. *Acta Neurologica Scandanavia* 87,234–238.

BEHAN PO & BAKHEIT AMO. (1991) Clinical spectrum of postviral fatigue syndrome. *British Medical Bulletin* (1991) Vol. 47, No 4, pp.793–808.

BEHAN PO & BEHAN WMH. (1988) Postviral fatigue syndrome. *CRC Critical Reviews in Neurobiology*, vol. 4, Issue 2, pp157–178.

BEHAN PO & HANIFFAH BAG. (1994) Chronic fatigue syndrome: a possible delayed hazard of pesticide exposure. *Clinical Infectious Diseases* 18 (Suppl 1):S54.

BEHAN PO. (1996) Chronic fatigue syndrome as a delayed reaction to chronic low dose organophosphate exposure. *Journal of Nutritional Medicine* (In press).

BIDARD JN, VIJVERBERG HPM, FRELIN C. (1984) Ciguatoxin is a novel type of Na+ channel toxin. *Journal of Biological Chemistry* **259:** 8353–8357.

BOU-HOLAIGAH I, ROWE PC, KAN J & CALKINS H. (1995) The relationship between neurally mediated hypotension and the chronic fatigue syndrome. *Journal of American Medical Association*, Vol. 274, No. 12, pp961.

BOUDOULAS H, TYSON CC, LEIGHTON RF & WILT SM. (1974) Myocardial lactate production in patients with angina-like chest pain and angiographically normal coronary arteries and left ventricle. *The American Journal of Cardiology*, Vol. 34, No 5., pp 501–505.

BURNET RB, YOAP BB, CHATTERTON BE & GAFFNEY RD (1996) Chronic fatigue syndrome: is total body potassium important? *Medical Journal of Australia* Vol 164, p 384.

CALVERT GM, HRYHORCZUK DO & LEIKIN JB. (1987) Treatment of ciguatera fish poisoning with amitriptyline and nifedipine. *Clinical Toxicology* 25(5), 423–428

CARRASCO L, PÉREZ L, IRURZUN A, LAMA J, MARTÍNEZ-ABARCA F, RODRÍGUEZ P. (1993) Modification of membrane permeability by animal viruses. *In: Regulation of Gene Expression in Animal viruses, pp283–303.* Carrasco L et al (eds). Plenum Press, New York.

DePASQUALE EE, NODY AC, DePUEY EG, et al. Quantitative rotational thallium-201 tomography for identifying and localizing coronary artery disease. *Circulation.* 1988;77:316–327.

DIAMOND GA, FORRESTER JS. Analysis of probability as an aid in the clinical diagnosis of coronary-artery disease. *NewEngland Journal of Medicine.* 1979;300:1350–1358.

DiNUBILE MJ, HOKAMA Y. (1995) The ciguatera poisoning syndrome from farm-raised salmon. *Annals of Internal Medicine* 1995;122:113–114.

ENGSTROM I, WALDENSTROM A, RONQUIST G. Ionophore A23187 reduces energy charge by enhanced ion pumping in suspended human erythrocytes. *Scandanavian Journal of Clinical Laboratory Investigation.* 1993; 53:239–46.

FRIEDBERG F. (1995) The stress/fatigue link in chronic fatigue syndrome. *In: Clinical management of chronic fatigue syndrome, pp147–152.* Klimas N & Patarca R (eds). The Haworth Medical Press, New York.

FUKUDA K, STRAUS SE, HICKIE I, SHARPE CM et al and the International Chronic Fatigue Syndrome Study Group. (1994) The chronic fatigue syndrome; a comprehensive approach to its definition and study. *Annals of Internal Medicine,* **121:** 959–963.

GILLESPIE N C, LEWIS RJ, PEARN JH, BOURKE ATC, HOLMES MJ, BOURKE JB & SHIELDS WJ. (1986) Ciguatera in Australia: occurrence, clinical features, pathophysiology and management. *Medical Journal of Australia,* Vol 145, pp584–590.

GOW JW, McGARRY F, BEHAN WMH, SIMPSON K & BEHAN PO. (1994) Molecular analysis of cell membrane ion channel function in chronic fatigue syndrome. *In: Abs. International Meeting on Chronic Fatigue Syndrome, Dublin, 1994.*

HANNAN WJ, COWEN SJ, PLESTER CE, FEAZRON KCH, deBEAU A. Comparison of bio-impedance spectroscopy and multi-frequency bio-impedance analysis for the assessment of extra-cellular and total body water in surgical patients. *Clinical Scientist.* 1995;89:651–8.

KAGAN B L, BALDWIN RL, MUNOZ D & WISNIESKI BJ. (1992) Formation of ion-permeable channels by tumor necrosis factor-α. *Science,* Vol. 255, pp1427–1430.

KLIMES I, MAYOU RA, PEARCE MJ, COLES L & FAGG JR. (1990) Psychological treatment for atypical non-cardiac chest pain: a controlled evaluation. *Psychological Medicine,* 1990, **20,** 605–611.

LANE RJM, BURGESS AP, FLINT J, RICCIO M & ARCHARD LC. (1995) Exercise responses and psychiatric disorder in chronic fatigue syndrome. *British Medical Journal,* **311:** 544–545.

LEIBEL RL, ROSENBAUM M, HIRSCH J. Changes in energy expenditure resulting from altered body weight (see comments) (published erratum appears in *New England Journal of Medicine* 1995 Aug 10;333(6):339). *New England Journal of Medicine* 1995;332:621–8.

MAJEED T & BEHAN PO. (1995) Clinical overview of chronic fatigue syndrome. *EOS—Journal of Immunology and Immunopharmacology.* Vol. XV, n. 1–2.

MARTINUSSEN HJ, WALDENSTROM A, RONQUIST G. Functional and biochemical effects of a K+ -ionophore on the isolated perfused rat heart. *Acta Physiologica Scandanavia.* 1993;147:221–5.

NELSON KM, WEINSIER RL, LONG CL, SCHUTZ Y. Prediction of resting energy expenditure from fat-free mass and fat mass. *American Journal of Clinical Nutrition.* 1992;56:848–56.

PEARN J. (1995) Ciguatera—A potent cause of the chronic fatigue syndrome. *EOS—Journal of Immunology and Immunopharmacology.* Vol. VX, n. 1–2.

RILEY MS, O'BRIEN CJ, McCLUSKEY DR, BELL NP & NICHOLLS DP. (1990) Aerobic work capacity in patients with chronic fatigue syndrome. *British Medical Journal* Vol. 301, pp 953–956.

SHARPE MC. (1991) A report—chronic fatigue syndrome: guidelines for research. *Journal of Royal Society of Medicine,* volume 84, pp118–121.

SOUSSI B, SCHERSTÉN T, WALDENSTRÖM A & RONQUIST G. (1993) Phosphocreatine turnover and pH balance in forearm muscle of patients with syndrome X. *The Lancet* Vol. 341: pp829 -830.

SYLVEN C. Sydrome X. *Journal of Internal Medicine* 1993:**234**: 431–433.

The facts about chronic fatigue syndrome. Meeting of the PHS CFS Interagency Coordinating Committee. US Department of Health and Human Services. CDC/NCID September, 28, 1993.

WALDENSTRÖM A, FOL=HLMAN J, ILBACK NG, RONQUIST G, HALLGREN R, GERDIN B. Coxsackie B3 myocarditis induces a decrease in energy charge and accumulation of hyaluronan in the mouse heart. *European Journal of Clinical Investigation.* 1993;23:277–82.

WALDENSTRÖM A, RONQUIST G, FOHLMAN J, GERDIN B & ILBACK N G. (1993) Ionophoric interaction with the myocyte sarcolemma : A new insight into the pathophysiology of degenerative myocardial disease. *Scandanavian Journal of Infectious Diseases—*Suppl. 88: 131–134.

WALDENSTRÖM A, RONQUIST G, LAGERQVIST B. Angina pectoris patients with normal coronary angiograms but abnormal thallium perfusion scan exhibit low myocardial and skeletal muscle energy charge. *Journal of Internal Medicine* . 1992;231:327–331.

WATSON WS. Total body potassium measurement—the effect of fallout from Chernobyl. *Clinical Physics & Physiological Measurement.* 1987;8:337–41.

7

CYTOKINE PATTERNS ASSOCIATED WITH CHRONIC FATIGUE SYNDROME

D. Sredni

Interdisciplinary Department
Bar Ilan University
Ramat Gan 52900, Israel

INTRODUCTION

As suggested by its name, the single main characteristic of chronic fatigue syndrome (CSF) is a severe long-lasting disabling fatigue. Both the etiology and pathophysiology of the disease are obscure. The fatigue may be accompanied by other chronic somatic symptoms of varying frequency and severity, and by flu-like symptoms (e.g. pharyngitis, adenopathy, low-grade fever, myalgia, arthralgia, headache) and neurophsychological manifestations (e.g. difficulty in concentrating, exercise intolerance, mental depression and a distrubance in sleep pattern (Holmes et al., 1988; Komaroff, 1993; McCluskey & Riley, 1992). Clinical examination and routine laboratory investigations generally yield no specific abnormalities.

Various theories have been proposed to explain the underlying pathophysiologic processes, but none of these has been fully proven. One is that certain infectious agents

Chronic Fatigue Syndrome, edited by Yehuda and Mostofsky
Plenum Press, New York, 1997

(including Epstein-Barr virus, human herpes virus 6, enteroviruses, and Brucella (Cluff, Trever, Imboden, & Canter, 1959; Evans, 1947; Gow et al., 1994; Holmes et al., 1987; Jones et al., 1985; Straus et al., 1985; Sumaya, 1991; Wakefield, Lloyd, Dwyer, Salahuddin, & Ablashi, 1988) may serve as triggers for an immunoregulatory abnormality that persists in these patients (Levy, 1994). Another theory ascribes CFS to enrivronmental factors, citing its simultaneous occurrence with sick building syndrome (Chester & Levine, 1994). Once an individual has been exposed to a triggering agent, cofactors may play a role in increasing host susceptibility to the developemnt of CFS (Kruesi, Dale, & Straus, 1989; Straus, Dale, Wright, & Metcalfe, 1988; Wessely & Powell, 1989; Wood, Bental, Gopfert, & Edwards, 1991).

The immune system is a readily accessible, sensitive indicator of environmental or physiological changes. Numerous studies have document evidence for immunological changes in CFS patients (Buchwald & Komaroff, 1991; Gupta & Vayuvegula, 1991; Klimas, Salvato, Morgan & Fletcher, 1990; Landay, Jessop, Lennett, and Levy, 1991; Patarca, Klimas, Lugtendorf, Antoni, & Fletcher, 1994; Prieto, Subir, Castilla, and Serrano, 1989). These studies have found decreased NK cell cytotoxicity, reduced mitogenic response of lymphocytes, increased expression of activation markers, reduced phagocytosis by monocytes, and altered cytokine production (Barker, Fujimura, Faden, Landay, & Levy, 1994; Caligiuri et al., 1987; Chao et al., 1991; Klimas et al., 1990; Landay et al., 1991; Lloyd, Hickie, Dwyer, & Wakefield, 1992). A recent study of CFS found a reduction of delayed-type hypersensitivity in 88% of the patients, providing very strong evidence for disordered T cell function. A statistically significant reduction in the absolute numbers of total T lymphocytes, helper/inducer T cells (CD4), and suppressor/cytotoxic T cells (CD8) was also observed in the patients (Lloyd, Wakefield, Boughton, & Dwyer, 1989).

With regard to humoral immunity, various investigators have reported that the serum IgG levels in patients with CFS are normal, elevated, or reduced in comparison with laboratory reference ranges. Nevertheless, it is clear from these reports that for the majority of CFS patients, serum levels of total IgG are normal. Findings from several case reports and one controlled study of a series of cases have suggested that serum levels of IgG subclasses (especially IgG1 and IgG3) may be reduced in patients with CFS. Although the mechanisms for the immunologic defects associated with CFS are unclear, such findings suggest that an immunoregulatory disorder may be involved in the pathophysiology of CFS.

The aim of this review is to present the recent findings on the immunological framework of CFS in general and the changes in cytokines in particular. The data presented suggest that the changes in cytokines may reveal biological markers of potential usefulness in the diagnosis, follow-up, and characterization of CFS.

RESULTS

1. Humoral Immunity in CFS

A defective humoral immune response to the infections thought to precipitate CFS may allow antigens to evade immune mechanisms (such as ADCC) crucial for the effective clearance of the agent from the host. Several works reported normal levels of CD20+ resting B cells, whereas other teams reported both increased and decreased levels (Borysiewicz et al., 1986; Buchwald & Komaroff, 1991; Klimas et al., 1990; Landay et al., 1991; Linde, Hammarstrom, & Smith, 1988). The proportion of CD5-bearing B cells was found to be increased or decreased (Klimas et al., 1990). When serum levels were tested, the total immunoglobulin G, A and M were typically within the normal reference range in CFS patients (Lloyd et al., 1989; Behan, Behan, & Bell, 1985). The immunoglobulin G (IgG) subclass distribution of antibodies generated in vivo in response to viral infections (including with

EBV, poliovirus, rubella and varicella-zoster virus) was predominantly restricted to the IgG1 and IgG3 subclasses (Skavril, 1986). IgG3 subclass deficiency has been associated with recurrent culture-negative upper respiratory symptoms and viral-like syndromes for which no specific infectious agent was found (Oxelius, Hanson, Bjorkander, Hammarstrom, & Sjoholm, 1986). Of potential interest, therefore, are several recent reports of patients with CFS with IgG subclass deficiencies.

A controlled study examining the serum levels of the IgG subclasses in CFS patients found that total IgG levels were within the laboratory reference range (7–16g/l) in all subjects. CFS patients had lower levels of IgG1, IgG2 and IgG3 when compared to the control subjects (Wakefield, Lloyd, & Brockman, 1990).

In terms of B cell function, spontaneous and mitogen-induced immunoglobulin synthesis is depressed in 10% of patients with CFS (Borysiewicz et al., 1986; Hamblin et al., 1983; Tosato, Straus, Henle, Pike, & Blaese, 1985). The latter decrease may be a result of an increased T cell suppression of immunoglobulin synthesis, because a similar effect is obtained in vitro when using normal allogeneic B cells (Tosato et al., 1985).

Despite the deficits in B cell function, stimulation with allergens provides differential lymphocyte responsiveness. Greater in vitro lymphocyte responses to specific allergens, greater baseline levels of lymphocyte incorporation of tritiated thymidine, and an increased number of IgE-bearing B lymphocytes have been reported.

Immunoglobulin production in vitro by peripheral blood mononuclear cells (PBMC) stimulated with pokeweed mitogen was normal in CFS patients (Chao et al., 1991), suggesting that the intrinsic capacity of T and B cells to cooperate in immunoglobulin production is not defective. This suggests that altered cytokine activity may play a role in B cell function in CFS. It is noteworthy in this respect that recent results show increases in the levels of circulating cytokines—IL-4 and IL-6—within the normal range, in a significant number of CFS patients, the significance of which will be disscussed later on under "Cytokines" (Olson, Kanaan, Gersuk, Kelley, & Jones, 1986; Olson, Kanaan, Kelley, & Jones, 1986).

2. Cellular Immunity in CFS

Natural Killer Cells (NK). Studies of cellular immunity in patients with CFS have initially focused on natural killer cells (NK). During acute viral infections, NK cells respond rapidly by cytolysis of infected cells. Several controlled studies have examined the number and function of NK cells in patients with CFS. They reported that the only cellular immune function in patients with CFS found to be consistently and significantly decreased was NK cells-mediated lysis, compared to that in healthy individuals. Moreover, those individuals with CFS in whom NK cell-mediated lysis was either elevated or normal were recovering from the illness. Thus, in agreement with the findings of other investigators, a decrease in NK cell-mediated lysis appears to be directly related to symptoms observed in CFS. The diminished lysis is not due to loss of NK cells among the PBMC, as has been reported by others (Caligiuri et al., 1987; Klimas et al., 1990; Morrison, Beha, & Behan, 1991), since the number of cells with NK phenotype among the PMC is normal. This decline in NK cell activity may be due in part to a reduction in NK cell target binding or to inefficient degranulation upon target-cell binding (Atkinson, Gerrard, Hildes, & Greenberg, 1990).

In a study of CFS using the older criteria for chronic active EBV infection, reduced NK cell function was found, especially when these cells were not separated from other lymphocytes and their cytokines (Kibler, Lucas, Hicks, Poulos, & Jones, 1985). A more recent study found a total reduction of NK cells with a specific reduction in the NKH1+T3- subset in CFS patients which represents the great majority of NK cells in normals, but a normal number of the NKH1+T3- subfraction cells which is a small fraction (about 20%) of NK cells in normals. Also the NK cells of CFS patients had low levels of killing against a variety of different targets. After activation with IL-2, the NK cells had increased activity against certain targets, but were still unable to lyse EBV-infected B cell targets. The NKH1+TK3- subfraction showed little activity in CFS patients, and most of the killing activity came form the NKH1+T3+ subfraction in these patients (Caligiuri et al., 1987).

The changes in NK cytotoxic activity found by most groups could be related to several findings: first, CD53+CD3- cells are the lymphoid subset with highest NK activity, and a decrease in their representation is expected to lower the value for the NK activity per effector cell; second, reduced NK activity may be associated with the finding of an impaired ability of lymphocytes from CFS patients to produce IL-2 and IFN-gamma in response to mitogenic stimuli, or in the ability of NK cells to respond to these lymphokines (Klimas et al., 1990; Kibler et al., 1985).

Furthermore, the lack of IFN-γ production in CFS patients may be responsible for the impaired activation of immunoregulatory circuits, which in turn facilitates the reactivation and progression of viral infections. In this respect, Lusso and associates described the prevention of intercellular spread of EBV mediated by the IFN released as a consequence of cellular response, and Borysiwicz et al. (1986) described normal NK cell activity but reduced EBV-specific cytotoxic T cell activity in their CFS patients (Lusso et al., 1987; Borysiewicz et al., 1986).

Monocytes. Prieto and coauthors found signifcant monocyte dysfunction in patients with CFS, such as a reduced display of vimentin, phagocytosis index, and surface expression of HLA-DR (Prieto et al., 1989). Recently, an increased expression of ICAM-1 in monocytes has been reported (Gupta & Vayuvegula, 1991). These changes in monocyte activity may affect the capability of the monocyte to produce monokines such as IL-10 and IL-12 that are important for balancing cellular and humoral immunity.

T Cells. Until recently, the functional activity of T cell subpopulations was associated with distinct surface phenotypes. Helper functions were associated with the CD4 surface marker and cytotoxic/suppressor functions with the CD8 marker. It is now known that helper T cells are found in both subsets and several studies have reported CD4+ cytotoxic and suppressor cells. Nevertheless, it has been established that both helper and cytotoxic/suppressor CD4+ T cells recognize antigen in association with class II MHC molecules, while CD8+ T cells, irrespective of their function, recognize antigen in association with class I MHC determinants (Naor, 1992).

Controlled studies of T cells in patients with CFS have included the enumeration of the number of peripheral blood T cell subsets by flow cytometry, an assessment of their proliferative capacity after stimulation in vitro by mitogens, and the in vivo evaluation of their capacity to respond to previously encountered antigens via delayed-type hypersensitivity (DTH) skin testing (Behan et al., 1985; Jones et al., 1985; Klimas et al., 1990; Landay et al., 1991; Lloyd et al., 1992; Lloyd et al., 1989; Straus et al., 1985).

Discrepant results have been reported in reference to CD4 and CD8 cell counts in CFS patients. Straus et al. (1985) reported a statistically higher percentage of CD4+ lymphocytes with normal numbers of CD8+ cells and CD4/CD8 raios; Jones et al. (1991) and Borysiewicz et al. (1986) and Landay et al. (1991) have found normal percentages of CD4+ and CD8+ cells as well as a normal CD4/CD8 raios; Lloyd et al. (1989) found decreased numbers of both CD4+ and CD8+ T cells; Buchwald and Komaroff (1991) found reduced numbers of CD8+ cells and higher than normal CD4/CD8 ratios; and Klimas et al. (1990) found that most CFS patients studied had a normal number of CD4+ cells and an elevated number of CD8+ cells that resulted in a decrease in the CD4/CD8 ratio. Decreased CD4/CD8 ratios in 2–100% of patients have been demonstrated by other investigators (Aoki, Usuda, Miyakashi, Tamura, & Herberman, 1987; Borysiewicz et al.,

1986; DuBois, 1986; Jones et al., 1985; Jones & Straus, 1987; Jones, 1991; Linde et al., 1988).

Klimas et al. (1990) found a decreased proportion of CD4+CD45RA+ cells, which are associated with suppressor/cytotoxic cell induction. Increased numbers of T cells expressing the activation marker CDw26, probably as a result of CD8+ actiavtion, have also been reported in CFS patients. In this respect, an increased proportion of CD8+ cells expression in the activation marker human leukocyte antigen (HLA)-DR (Klimas et al., 1990; Landay et al., 1991) has been reported in CFS patients, whereas normal proportions of CD4+ T cells co-expressing the HLA-DR marker or the IL-2 receptor (CD25) were found in one study. In a recent study CD11b on CD8+ cells was found to be significantly decreased in CFS patients. These conflicting results may be associated with the fluctuations in clinical manifestations of these patients.

In contrast to the previous studies, the capacity of peripheral blood T cells to proliferate in response to mitogen has been shown to be impaired in all five controlled studies which included adequate numbers of patients (Behan et al., 1985; Klimas et al., 1990; Lloyd et al., 1992; Skavril, 1986; Straus et al., 1985). Impaired lymphocyte responsiveness to mitogen has been reported to be prevalent in patients with major depression (Hickie, Silove, Hickie, Wakefield, & Lloyd, 1990). A recent study has shown that lymphocyte proliferation in response to PHA was significantly reduced in CFS patients compared to either healthy controls or to subjects with major depression (Lloyd et al., 1992).

The capacity to mount a recall or DTH response in vivo to an intradermally injected antigen depends on prior exposure to the antigen and on effective T cells and macrophage function. DTH skin responses have been used to assess the cell-mediated immune function in CFS patients and healthy controls (Behan et al., 1985; Klimas et al., 1990; Lloyd et al., 1992; Skavril, 1986; Straus et al., 1985).

Four studies used a commercially available kit employing seven test antigens and a glycerin control (Multitest CMI, Merieux, France). The rates of cutaneous anergy in CFS patients ranged from 21–54% and in the controls from 0–15%. A confirmation of these results was found in a report comparing healthy controls, patients with major depression, and CFS patients—in the latter group of which skin allergy was 30–50%, while in the first two it was only 10% (Lloyd, Hickie, Boughton, Spencer, & Wakefield, 1990; Lloyd et al., 1992; Murdoch, 1988; Skavril, 1986; Straus et al., 1985).

3. Cytokines

Cytokines are protein cell regulators produced by a wide range of cells that play important roles in many physiological responses. They are low-molecular-weight proteins invloved in immunity and inflammation.

Most cytokines have a variety of effects on many different cells but despite this overlap, cytokine functions are not identical. Different cytokines induce different subsets of T cells or have different effects on proliferation within a particular subset. Thus, there appears to be a very complex network of interactions within the immune system (Mosmann, 1991). Mosmann believes that this complexity is essential for overcoming the various defense strategies of microorganisms (Table 1).

In 1986 Mosmann et al. identified two distinct subsets of murine CD4+ Th cell clones showing different patterns of cytokine production and effector function (Mosmann, Chervinshi, Bond, Giedlin, & Coffman, 1986). Th1 cells secrete interleukin-2 (1L-2) and interferon (IFNγ) and are the principal effectors of cell-mediated immunity against intracellular microbes and of delayed-type hypersensitivity reactions. Murine Th1 cells can also stimulate production of antibodies of the IgG2a class, which are effective at activating complement and opsonizing antigens for phagocytosis. Th2 cells, on the other hand, produce IL-4 and IL-6, which stimulate IgE and IgG1 antibody production, IL-5,

Table 1. Summary of cytokine functions

Cytokine	Cellular sources	Biological activity
IL-1α	monocytes/macrophages endothelial and neuronal cells keratinocytes fibroblasts T and B cells	Activates T and B cells, endothelial cells, pyrogenic, acute-phase response; hematopoiesis.
IL-1β	monocytes/macrophages endothelial and neuronal cells keratinocytes fibroblasts T and B cells	Activates T and B cells, endothelial cells, pyrogenic, acute-phase response; hematopoiesis.
IL-2	T cells	function; Enhances cytolytic activity of NK cells and CTL; Promotes proliferation and Ig secretion B cells.
IL-4	T cells mast cells basophils BM stroma cells	Induces Th2 cell differentiation; Induces proliferation and differentiation of B cells; Inhibits Il-2 and IFNγ-induced activities; Inhibits IL-12 production.
IL-6	T cells monocytes/macrophages fibroblasts hepatocytes endothelial and neuronal cells	Growth and differentiation of B and T cells and other cells; Major role in mediation of inflammation immune response initiated by infection and injury.
IL-10	T and B cells monocytes/macrophages	Suppresses macrophage function and IL-12 production; Suppresses proliferation and cytokine production by activated T cells; Inhibits macrophage-derived proinflammatory cytokines; Enhances B cell proliferation and differentiation.
IL-12	B cells	Stimulates growth and cytotoxic activity of NK and T monocytes/macrophages cells; Necessary for Th1 induction;
IFNγ	T cells; NK cells	Requisite for induction of Th1 cells; Stimulates macrophage activity, CTL, and NK cells; Inhibits IL-4 activities; Enhances IL-12 production.
TNFα	monocytes	Cytotoxic, T-cell activation, antitumor, pyrogenic, septic shock.
TGFβ	platelets	Fibroblast growth and collagen production inhibition of cytokine

an eosinophil-activating factor, IL-10, which together with IL-4 inhibits macrophage functions. There is evidence that human CD4+ T cells have cytokine patterns and functions comparable to those that exist in mice (Bloom, Salgame, & Diamond, 1992). Th1 cytokines are generally elevated in successful responses to many intracellular pathogens, while Th2 cytokines are elevated in allergic diseases and helminth infections. Th2 cells stimulate mast cells, eosinophils and IgE antibodies. Th1 cells increase the ability of macrophages to kill intracellular and extracellular pathogens and also mediate delayed-type hypersensitivity (DTH) reactions. Th1 and Th2 cells play different roles not only in protection against exogenous antigens but also in immunopathology (Romagnani, 1992). Therefore, each T helper subset induces and regulates effector functions targeted at different antigens and pathogens. Recent studies suggest that the immune reponse to infection is in fact regulated by the balance between Th1 and Th2 cytokines. These two pathways are often mutually exclusive, the one resulting in protection and to the other in progression of a disease (Cox & Liew, 1992).

It would seem, therefore, that in CFS patients the cytokine pattern may underlie several of the pathological manifestations.

A. Proinflammatory Cytokines in CFS. Interleukin-1 (IL-1). Isolation of cDNA clones has shown that there are two forms—IL-1α and IL-1β, both of which bind to the same receptor and have identical biological properties. IL-1 is the principal mediator of inflammatory responses. During inflammation, injury, immunolgoical challenge or infection, IL-1α and IL-1β are produced and can affect the pathogenesis of disease thanks to their multiple biological properties. IL-1 is produced by many different cells, including macrophages, endothelial cells, B cells, fibrobalsts, epithelial cells, astrocytes, and osteoblasts (Dinarello, 1987). One of the most important actions of IL-1 is its induction of other cytokines and it appears to be part of a network of cytokines with self-regulating and self-

suppressing properties (Ghezzi & Dinarello, 1988). Increased production of IL-1β in vitro by PBMC in response
to Lipopolysaccaride (LPS) in CFS patients was found by
Chao et al. (1991). In contrast, IL-1 production was not
found to be increased in an earlier study (Morte, Castilla,
Civiera, Serrano, & Prieto, 1989). Moreover, recent studies
using a whole blood culture system that does not require
isolation of PBMC and probably more closely resembles the
in vivo situation (Drenth et al., 1995) shows that in contrast to the results of Chao et al. (1991) there was a significant decrease in IL-1β proudction after LPS stimuation of
peripheral blood cells. The difference in the results of
these two studies may be due to the fact that the cells
were separated and no autologous plasma was added in
the first study. Taken together we may hypothesize that
plasma factors that inhibit cytokine production occur in
CFS. Several inhibitory factors could be responsible for
this. An increased concentration of TGF-β, as found by
Chao et al. (1991), could explain the results, as TGF-β is
known to inhibit the production of proinflammatory cytokines.

Tumor Necrosis Factor-Alpha (TNFα). TNFα is a 17kDa
protein. Although cells from the monocyte/macrophage
lineage have been the most extensively studied for TNFα
production, and are taken to be its principal source in
vivo, a number of other cells are capable of secreting it as
well. These include lymphoyctes, mast cells, basophils,
eosinophils, NK cells, B cells, T cells and astrocytes. The
biological effects of TNFα have been studied in isolated tissue culture and organ perfusion systems. From these
there appears to be a general consensus that TNFα is a
key mediator of inflammation and the mammalian hosts's
response to injury or invasion by microbes, parasites, or
neoplasia, in the intact organism, and in some isolated organ system. Early studies showed that in a small percent
of CFS patients there is an elevation in the serum level of
TNFα (Lloyd, Wakefield, & Hickie, 1993). But a recent
study in endotoxin-stimulated ex-vivo production of TNFα

using whole blood culture system showed that it was significantly lower in CFS patients compared to healthy controls. The method used to measure cytokine production may reflect the in vivo situation more closely since manipulation, prestimulation and possible selection of PMNC are minimized and the role of plasma factors are included, as described earlier with respect to IL-1 (Swanink et al., 1996).

B. Cytokines Produced by Th1 Cells. Interleukin -2 (IL-2). IL-2 was first discovered through its activity as a T cell growth factor. It is secreted and synthesized by T cells after activation by antigen or mitogen and plays a central role in T cell division. Not only does IL-2 act as an autocrine growth factor, it also induces T cells cytotoxicity and natural killer cell activity (O'Garra, 1989). Early studies have shown that serum levels of IL-2 were found to be strikingly elevated in CFS patients compared to healthy controls (Cheney, Dorman, & Bell, 1989), but decreased levels of IL-2 were reported in different studies (Kibler et al., 1985; Gold et al., 1990). Recent studies also have shown that CFS patietns had elevated levels of sIL-2R. This result is consistent with the reduced levels of IL-2 and decreased levels of NK cytotoxic activity found in several studies (Peterson et al., 1994).

Interferon-Gamma (IFN-γ). IFN-γ belongs to the network of cytokines that are involved in the contorl of cellular function and become actively engaged in host defense during infection. IFNγ is produced during an immune response by antigen-specific T cells and NK cells recruited by IL-2 and IL-12. Its regulatory effects include the activation of macrophages to enhance their phagocytosis and tumor killing capability as well as activation and growth enhancement of CTL an NK cells (Morris, 1988; O'Garra, 1989).

IFNγ plays a major role in the control of immunoglobulin isotypes produced during an immune response. In the mouse IgG2a is enhanced with suppression of other IgG isotypes and IgE (Snapper & Paul, 1987; Finkelman, Katona, Mosmann, & Coffman, 1987). IgG2a is very effective at fixing complement and promoting NK cell mediated killing so that IFNγ promotes the ability of the humoral immune system to destroy microbial pathogens. IFNγ inhibits most of the activities induced by Th2 cells and appears to be a requisite factor for the induction of the Th1 subset (Scott, 1993). Several groups have found decreased IFNγ production on mitogenic stimulation of peripheral blood mononuclear cells from CFS patients (Peterson et al., 1994).

In summary, the capacity for an effective cellular response to specific agents, especially involving cytotoxic T cells and NK cells, may be reduced because of overall T helper suppression or because of lack of specific helper factors. This reduced reactivity may be reflected in the decreased capacity to mount delayed hypersensitivity responses in CFS patients.

C. Cytokines Produced by Th2 Cells. Interleukin-4 (IL-4). IL-4 was identified for its ability to induce activated mouse B lymphocytes to proliferate and to secrete immunoglobulins. IL-4 is produced by T cells, mast cells, and basophils (Sher et al., 1992), and is an important factor in the clonal expansion of antigen-specific B cells. IL-4 enhances IgE synthesis in both the mouse (Coffman et al., 1986) and human (Del Prete et al., 1988), IgG1 in murine B cells (Scott, 1993), and IgG4 in human cells (Lundgren et al., 1989).

It would appear that IL-4 modulates humoral responses to different antigenic stimuli. IL-4 contributes to negative immune regulation by its ability to reduce IL-2 receptors thus inhibiting some IL-2-induced activities. These include the IL-2-induced generation of NK cells and IFNγ enhanced activities, including the activation of macrophages and their anitmicrobial activity (O'Garra, 1989). IL-4 can also block macrophage nitric oxide generation necessary for the killing of intracellular parasites (Modlin & Nutman, 1993).

Recent studies have found elevation within the normal range in the levels of circulating IL-4 in a significant number of CFS patients (Morris, 1988). The increase in IL-4 levels may be associated with the allergies seen in high frequency (70%) in CFS patients (Klimas et al., 1990; Straus et al., 1988). It is also noteworthy that many of the effects of IL-4 are antagonized by IFNγ whose production is reduced in activated T cells from CFS patients. Moreover, upregulation of IL-4 may activate CD5-bearing B cells that are found in increased levels in a significant number of CFS patients (Klimas et al., 1990).

Interleukin-6 (IL-6). IL-6 is produced by both hemopoietic and nonhemopoietic cells and induces immunoglobulin secretion in both preactivated murine and human B cells and therefore induces the final maturation of B cells into high-rate Ig-secreting cells (O'Garra, 1989). IL-6 activity is not restricted to B cells and appears to be a key member of the cytokine network being expressed at high levels by many cell types both constitutively or after activation and interacts with many targets (Tovey et al., 1988; Wong & Clark, 1988).

Serum levels of IL-6 were found to increase in signficant numbers of CFS patients. Excessive IL-6 production has been associated with polyclonal B cell activation, resulting in hypergammaglobulinemia and autoantibody production (Van Snick, 1990). IL-6 may contribute to activation of CD5-bearing B cells that are found in increased proportion in a significant number of CFS patients (Klimas et al., 1990).

D. Anti-Inflammatory Cytokines. Transforming Growth Factor beta (TGFβ). There is considerable evidence for an immunomodualory role of TGFβ and its function as a potent differentiation modulating and immunosuppressive agent (Kehrl, Thevenin, Rieckmann, & Fauci, 1991; Roberts & Sporn, 1990; Ruscetti, Vanesio, Ochoa, & Ontaldo, 1993; Walh et al, 1988). In culture, most cells of the immune system, such as lymphoyctes and monocytes, synthesize TGFβ

(Kehrl et al., 1991). The TGFβ released by these cells is mostly latent, suggesting that activation of the latent complex is required before TGFβ can exert its effect. Treatment of lymphoyctes and monocytes with TGFβ results in a large array of biological responsess, dependent on the cell type and its differentiation state. One of the most potent activities of TGFβ on lymphocytes is its antiproliferative effect. TGFβ inhibits the proliferation of T lymhpyctes, B lymphocytes, thymocytes, large granular lymphocytes, NK cells, and LAK cells (Kehrl, Roberts, et al., 1986; Kehrl, Wakefiled, et al., 1986; Kehrl et al., 1991; Kuppner, Hamou, Bodmer, Fontanta, & De Tribolet, 1988; Ortaldo et al., 1991; Ristow, 1986; Rook et al., 1986; Wahl et al., 1988). In monocytes TGFβ inhibits the effect and/or the production of IFNγ, TNFα and IL-1 (Kehrl et al., 1991; Roberts & Sporn, 1990). Several studies have shown consistently elevated serum levels of TGFβ in patients with CFS (Chao et al., 1991; MacDonald et al., 1996). Given the immunosuppressive role of TGFβ (Schluesener & Lider, 1989; Walh, McCartney-Francis, & Mergenhagen, 1989), significantly higher serum TGFβ levels in CFS patients could be explaind by the abnormal T lymphocytes and NK fucntions detected in CFS patients, and also account for the lower serum IgG levels detected in these patients (Chao et al., 1991).

Interleukin-10 (IL-10). IL-10 plays a major role in suppressing immune and inflammatory responses. It is produced by T cells, including human Th0, Th1 and Th2 cells. B cells, and monocytes/macrophages after activation (De Waal Malefyt, Yssel, Roncarolo, Spits, & De Vries, 1992). It is produced at a relatively late stage of activation, indicating a regulatory role in the latter stages of the immune response (Yssel et al., 1992).

Human IL-10 significantly reduces the proliferation and production of cytokines of Th1 clones exposed to specific antigen and PHA (Del Prete et al., 1988). IL-10 contributes to the suppression of IFNγ-induced macrophage-mediated immune destruction of pathogens (De Waal Malefyt et al., 1993). In clinical situations, IL-10 activity may not be desirable because it could result in the downregulation of the IFNγ-induced antiviral activity of CTLs and NK cells (Howard & O'Garra, 1992).

IL-10 is a potent growth and differentiation factor for activated human B cells and therefore may play an important role in the amplification of the humoral immune response (Rousset et al., 1992). The synthesis of monocyte-derived proinflammatory cytokines, including IL-1α and IL-6 are inhibited by IL-10, which also enhances the production of IL-1 receptor antagonist so that this cytokine dampens immune proliferation and inflammatory responses (De Waal Malefyt et al., 1993). Therefore, it woud appear that IL-10 plays a role in diminishing DTH reactions and other Th1 cell-mediated responses.

Preliminary results in our laboratory show that some patients had increased levels of IL-10 after MNC were activated with LPS as compared to controls. These results dovetail with the recent findings that TGFβ enhances IL-10 production ability in macrophages (Maeda et al., 1995).

It would seem that the increase in IL-10 levels in CFS patients is the result of higher levels of TGFγ. Elevated IL-10 levels are known to inhibit cytokine production by Th1 cells, such as IL-2, IFNγ, which may account for the decrease in NK activity in these patients. In addition, IL-10 may also induce an increase in Th2 cytokines, which may explain the increase in allergies and in high IgE levels in CFS patients.

Similarly changes in IL-10 levels may account for the reduction or absence of DTH skin testing responses in CFS patients. Interestingly, it was recently found that administration of IL-10 to the central nervous system (CNS) of rats reduces spontaneous non-REM sleep in otherwise normal animals. These results implicate IL-10 in the pathophysiology of CFS (Opp, Smith, & Hughes, 1995).

DISCUSSION AND CONCLUSION

The pathophysiology of CFS remains unknown. However, circumstantial evidence suggests that the condition may result from a disordered immune response to a precipitating infection or antigenic challenge.

The data presented in the present review indicate that CFS is associated with immune abnormalitites that can account for many of its characteristic symptoms. With regard to humoral immunity, though discrepant serum IgG levels were reported, it seems clear that serum levels of total IgG were normal in the majority of CFS patients, whereas serum levels of IgG subclasses (especially IgG1 and IgG3) were reduced.

In controlled studies of T cells in CFS patients the three most prominent and apparently reproducible findings were: 1) imparied lymphocyte proliferation in response to stimulation by mitogens; 2) impaired NK cytotoxicity against the K562 erythroleukemia cells line; 3) impaired cell-mediated immune function in vivo suggested by the increased number of reduced or absent DTH skin testing responses.

The regulation of a cellular and humoral immune response to antigen is critically dependent on the activity of soluble proteins—cytokines—which function as intercellular messengers. Although essential for effective immunity, cytokines may also directly produce clinical symptoms such as profound fatigue, neuropsychiatric symptoms and sleep disorders all of which are reminiscent of CFS. There are however numerous factors which may contribute to difficulties in detecting the presence and activity of cytokines CFS. In addition, different assay systems for cytokine detection were used in each of the reported studies possibly accounting for the wide variability of results. A further difficulty is that many of the cytokines have naturally occurring inhibitors (produced in response to the same stimuli) which may interfere with the detection of the particular cytokine in body fluids.

The discovery of two polarized forms of effector specific immune response has been of great improtance not only for understanding the mechanisms of protection against exogenous offending agents, but also for our knowledge of the pathogenesis of different human diseases. Several pathophysiological conditions have indeed been suspected to results from the dominant Th1 or Th2-type responses. Looking over the many studies on cytokine production in CFS patients, the overall picture is one in where the Th1 cytokines—IL-2 and IFNγ—were decreased compared to the Th2 cytokines—IL-4 and IL-6—which were increased or found to be in the normal range.

These findings suggest that in CFS patients there is a trend towards Th2 cell type differentiation which would also explain the latest results showing a decrease in inflammatory cytokines such as IL-1 and TNFα in these patients. This may be the outcome of the elevated levels of TGFβ that also induces enhanced production of IL-10 in macrophages, suggesting a new aspect of the role of TGFβ in the immune system (Maeda & Shiraishi, 1996). Figure 1 shows a hypothetical summary of cytokine production in CFS.

Some human beings have a genetic predisposition to be triggered by an agent or event that will cause an immune dysequilibrium, which would mean an increase in TGFβ or in IL-10. The increase in these will cause a decrease in IL-1,TNFα and in IL-12. This in turn will diminish NK cell activity, and lowered IFNγ levels would prevent differentiation of Th0 into Th1 which would further decrease the levels of factors produced by these cells—IL-2 and IFNγ, since IL-10 is known to directly inhibit Th1 cells from producing these cytokines. These findings may explain the decrease in cellular immunity including reduced lymphocyte proliferation in response to stimulation by mitogens, the impaired activity of NK cells and the reduced or absence of DTH skin test responses of patients with CFS. On the other hand, it would also explain the upregulation of IL-4, found to be elevated in a significant number of CFS patients (Peterson et al., 1994). They also shed light on the allergies associated with CFS—about 65% of the patients having a premorbid history of inhalant, food, or drug allergies (Romagnani, 1992). CFS patients suffer from flu-like symptoms that could be the result of the increase in IL-4 as shown by a recent clinical trial in which patient

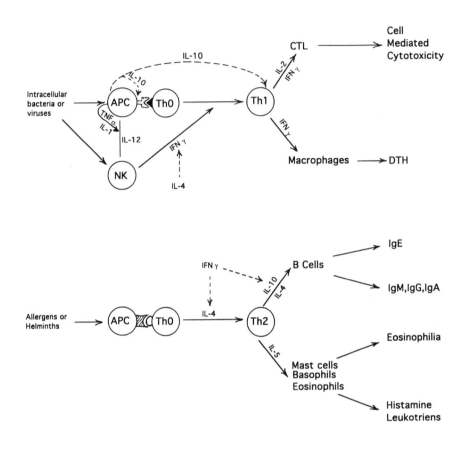

Figure 1. Th1 and Th2 induction and regulation (—— stimulation, ---- inhibition).

toxicity consisted primarily of flu-like symptoms with fatigue, somnolence, fever and myalgias.

Sleep laboratory research has demonstrated that patients with CFS have a specific lack of normal deep, non-REM, sleep. This is manifested clinically by initial and middle insomnia, restless sleep, night sweats, nonrestorative sleep, and nightmares, and during investigation by intrusive alpha EEG activity during non-REM sleep

(Moldofsky, 1993; Morriss et al., 1993). In one recent study, polysomnography revealed that 10 (62.5%) of 16 patients with CFS had clinically relevant sleep abnormalities (Krupp, Jandorf, Coyle, & Mendelson, 1993). These could be the result of the elevated levels of IL-10 since it was found that administration of IL-10 into the CNS of rats reduces spontaneous NREM sleep in otherwise normal animals thus providing additional support for the hypothesis that cytokines are involved in the regulation of sleep.

In summary we hypothesize that CFS involves an immunologic imbalance characterized by a predominance in TH2. Probably no single theory can account for the complex phenomena observed in CFS patients—a multifactorial etiology is more likely (Lewis & Wessely, 1992). But we believe that the role of changes in cytokine production levels in this multifactorial etiology of CFS deserves further investigation.

REFERENCES

Aoki, T., Usuda, Y., Miyakashi, H., Tamura, K., & Herberman, R. B. (1987). Low natural killer syndrome: clinical and immunologic features. *Natural Immunity & Cell Growth Regulation, 6*, 116–128.

Atkinson, E. A., Gerrard, J. M., Hildes, G. E., & Greenberg, A .H. (1990). Studies of the mechanism of natural killer degranulation and cytotoxicity. *Journal of Leukocyte Biology, 47*, 39–48.

Barker, E., Fujimura, S. F., Faden, M. B., Landay, A. L., & Levy, J. A. (1994). Immunologic abnormalities associated with chronic fatigue syndrome. *Clinical and Infectious Diseases,18(1),* S136-S141.

Behan, P. O., Behan, W. M., & Bell, E. J. (1985). The postviral fatigue syndrome—an analysis of the findings in 50 cases. *Journal of Infections, 10*, 211–222.

Bloom, B. R., Salgame, P., & Diamond, B. (1992). Revisiting and revising suppresson T cells. *Immunology Today,13*, 131–136.

Borysiewicz, L. K., Haworth, S. J., Cohen, J., Mundin, J., Rickinson, A., & Sissons, J. G. (1986). Epstein-Barr virus—specific immune defects in patients with persistent symptoms following infectious mononucleosis. *Quarterly Journal of Medicine, 58*, 111–121.

Buchwald, D., & Komaroff, A. L. (1991). Review of laboratory findings for patients with chronic fatigue syndrome. *Review of Infectious Diseases, 13(1),* S12-S18.

Caligiuri, M., Murray, C., Buchwald, D., Levine, H., Cheney, P., Peterson, D., Komaroff, A. L., & Ritz, J. (1987). Phenotypic and functional deficiency of natural killer cells in patients with chronic fatigue syndrome. *Journal of Immunology, 139*, 3306–3313.

Chao, C. C., Janoff, E. N., Hu, S. X., Thomas, K., Galagher, M., Tsang, M., & Peterson, P. K. (1991). Altered cytokine release in peripheral blood mononuclear cell cultures from patients with the chronic fatigue syndrome. *Cytokine, 3*, 292–298.

Cheney, P. R., Dorman, S. E., & Bell, D. S. (1989). Interleukin-2 and the chronic fatigue syndrome (letter). *Annals of Internal Medicine, 110*, 321.

Chester, A. C., & Levine, P. H. (1994). Concurrent sick building syndrome and chronic fatigue syndrome: epidemic neuromyasthenia revisited. *Clinical and Infectious Diseases, 18(1)*, S43-S48.

Cluff, L. E., Trever, R. W., Imboden, J. B., & Canter, A. (1959). Brucellosis II. Medical aspects of delayed convalescence. *Archive of Internal Medicine, 103*, 398–405.

Coffman, R. L., Ohara, J., Bond, M. W., Carty, J., Zlotnik, A., & Paul, W. E. (1986). B cell stimulatory factor-1 enhances the IgE response of Lipopolysaccharide-activated B cells. *Journal of Immunology, 136*, 4538–4541.

Cox, F. E. G. , & Liew, F. Y. (1992). T-cell subsets and cytokines in parasitic infections. *Immunology Today, 13*, 445–448.

De Waal Malefyt, R., Yssel, H., Roncarolo, M. G., Spits, H., & de Vries, J. E. (1992). Interleukin-10. *Current Opinion in Immunology, 4*, 314–320.

De Waal Malefyt, R., Yssel, H., & de Vries, J. E. (1993). Direct effects of IL-10 on subsets of human CD4+ T cell clones and resting T cells. Specific inhibition of IL-2 production and proliferation. *Journal of Immunology, 150(11)*, 4754–4765.

Del Prete, G., Maggi, E., Parronchi, P., Chretiem, A., Tiri, D., Macchia, H., Ricci, J., Banchereau, J., de Vries, J. E., & Romagnani, S. (1988). IL-4 is an essential factor for the IgE synthesis induced in vitro by human T cell clones and their supernatants. *Journal of Immunology, 140*, 4193–4198.

Dinarello, C. A. (1987). The biology of interleukin 1 and comparison to tumor necrosis factor. *Immunology Letters, 16*, 227–232.

Drenth, J. P. H., van Hum, S. H. M., van Deuren, M., Pesman, G. J., van der Ven-Jongekrijg, J., & van der Meer, J. W. M. (1995). Endurance run increases circulating IL-6 and IL-1RA but down-regulates ex vivo TNFα and IL-1β production. *Journal of Applied Physiology, 79*, 1497–1503.

Du Bois, R. E. (1986). Gamma globulin therapy for chronic mononucleosis syndrome. *AIDS Research and Human Retroviruses, 2(1)*, S191-S195.

Evans, A. C. (1947). Brucellosis in the United States. *American Journal of Public Health, 37*, 139–151.

Finkelman, F. D., Katona, I. M., Mosmann, T. R., & Coffman, R. L. (1988). IFN-γ regulates the isotypes of Ig secreted during in vivo humoral immune responses. *Journal of Immunology, 140*, 1022–1027.

Ghezzi, P., & Dinarello, C. A. (1988). IL-1 induces IL-1. III. Specific inhibition of IL-1 production by IFNγ. *Journal of Immunology, 140*, 4238–4244.

Gold, D., Bowden, R., Sixbey, J., Riggs, R., Katon, W. J., Ashley, R., Obrigewitch, R. M., & Corey, L. (1990). Chronic fatigue. A prospective clinical and virolgoic study. *Journal of the American Medical Association, 264*, 48–53.

Gow, J. W., Behan, W. M. H., Simpson, K., McGarry, F., Keir S., & Behan, P. O. (1994). Studies on enterovirus in patients with chronic fatigue syndrome. *Clinical and Infectious Diseases, 18(1)*, S126-S129.

Gupta, S., Vayuvegula, B. A. (1991). A comprehensive immunological analysis in chronic fatigue syndrome. *Scandinavian Journal of Immunology, 33*, 319–327.

Hamblin, T. J., Hussain, J., Akbar, A. N., Tang, Y.C., Smith, J. L., & Jones, D. B. (1983). Immunogical reason for chronic ill health after infectious mononucleosis. *British Medical Journal, 287*, 85–88.

Hickie, I., Silove, D., Hickie, C., Wakefield, D., & Lloyd, A. (1990). Is there signficant immune dysfunction in depressvie disorders? *Psychological Medicine, 20*, 755–761.

Holmes, G. P., Kaplan, J. E., Stewart, J. A., Hunt, B., Pinsky, P. F., & Schonberger, L. B. (1987). A cluster of patients with a chronic mononucleosis-like syndrome. *Journal of the American Medical Association, 257*, 2297–2302.

Holmes, G. P., Kaplan, J. E., Gantz, N. M., Komaroff, A. L., Schonberger, L. B., Straus, S. E., Jones, J. F., Du Bois, R. E., & Cunningham-Rundles, C. (1988). Chronic fatigue syndrome: a working case definition. *Annals Internal Medicine, 108*, 387–389.

Howard, M., & O'Garra, A. (1992). Biological properties of interleukin *Immunology Today, 13*, 198–200.

Jones, J. F., Ray, G., Minnich, L. L., Hicks, M. J., Kibler, R., & Lucas, D. O. (1985). Evidence for active Epstein-Barr virus infection in patients with persistent, unexplained illnesses: elevated anti-early antigen antibodies. *Annals of Internal Medicine, 102*, 1–7.

Jones, J. F., & Straus, S. E. (1987). Chronic Epstein-Barr virus infection. *Annual Review of Medicine, 38*, 195–209.

Jones, J. (1991). Serologic and immunologic responses in chronic fatigue syndrome with emphasis on the Epstein-Barr virus. *Review of Infectious Diseases, 13(1)*, S26-S31.

Kehrl, J. H., Roberts, A. B., Wakefield, L. M., Jakowlew, S., Sporn, M. B., & Fauci, A. S. (1986). Transforming growth factor-β is an important immunomodulatory protein for human B lymphocytes. *Journal of Immunology, 137*, 3855–3860.

Kehrl, J. H., Wakefield, L. M., Roberts, A. B., Jakowlew, S., Alvarez-Mon, M., Derynck, R., Sporn, M. B., & Fauci, A. S. (1986). Production of transforming growth factor-β by human B lymphocytes and its potential role in the regulation of T cell growth. *Journal of Experimental Medicine, 163*, 1037–1050.

Kehrl, J. H., Thevenin, C., Rieckmann, R., & Fauci, A. S. (1991). Transforming growth factor-β suppressed human B lymphocyte Ig production by inhibiting synthesis and the switch from the membrane form to the secreted form of Ig mRNA. *Journal of Immunology, 146*, 4016–4022.

Kibler, R., Lucas, D. O., Hicks, M. H., Poulos, B. T., & Jones, J. F. (1985). Immune function in chronic active Epstein-Barr virus infection. *Journal of Clinical Immunology, 5*, 46–54.

Klimas, N. G., Salvato, F. R., Morgan, R., & Fletcher, M. A. (1990). Immunologic abnormalities in chronic fatigue syndrome. *Journal of Clinical Microbiology, 28*, 1403–1410.

Komaroff, A. L., (1993). Clinical presentation of chronic fatigue syndrome. *Ciba Foundation Symposium, 173*, 43–54, Discussion: 54–61.

Kruesi, M. J. P., Dale, J., & Straus, S. E. (1989). Psychiatric diagnoses in patients who have chronic fatigue syndrome. *Journal of Clinical Psychiatry, 50*, 53–56.

Krupp, L. B., Jandorf, L., Coyle, P. K., & Mendelson, W. B. (1993). Sleep disturbance in chronic fatigue syndrome. *Journal of Psychosomatic Research, 37*, 325–331.

Kuppner, M. C., Hamou, M. F., Bodmer, S., Fontanta, A., & De Tribolet, N. (1988). The glioblastoma-derived T-cell suppressor factor/transforming growth factor beta$_2$ inhibits the generation of lymphokine-activated killer (LAK) cells. *International Journal of Cancer, 42*, 562–567.

Landay, A. L., Jessop, C., Lennett, E. T., & Levy, J. A. (1991). Chronic fatigue syndrome: clinical condition associated with immune activation. *Lancet, 338*, 702–712.

Levy, J. A. (1994). Part III: Viral studies of chronic fatigue syndrome. Introduction. *Clinical Infectious Disease, 18(1)*, 117–120.

Lewis, G., & Wessely, S. (1992). The epidemiology of fatigue: more questions than answers. *Journal of Epidemiology and Community Health, 46*, 92–97.

Linde, A., Hammarstrom, L., & Smith, C. I. E. (1988). IgG subclass deficiency and chronic fatigue syndrome (letter). *Lancet, 1*, 885–886.

Linde, A., Andersson, B., Svenson, S. B., Ahrne, H., Carlsson, M., Forsberg, P., Hugo, H., Karstorp, A., Lenkei, R., & Lindwall, A. (1992).

Serum levels of lymphokines and soluble cellular receptors in primary Epstien-Barr virus infection and in patients with chronic fatigue syndrome. *Journal of Infectious Diseases, 165,* 994–1000.

Lloyd, A. R., Wakefield, D., Boughton, C. R., & Dwyer, J. M. (1989). Immunological abnormalities in chronic fatigue syndrome. *Medical Journal of Ausralia,151,* 122–124.

Lloyd, A. R., Hickie, I., Boughton, C. R., Speneer, O., & Wakefield, D. (1990). The prevalence of chronic fatigue syndrome in an Australian population. *Medical Journal of Australia, 153,* 522–528.

Lloyd, A., Hickie, C., Dwyer, J., & Wakefield, D. (1992). Cell-mediated immunity in patients with chronic fatigue syndrome, healthy control subjects and patients with major depression. *Clinical and Experimental Immunology, 87,* 76–79.

Lloyd, A. R., Wakefield, D., & Hickie, I. (1993). Immunity and the pathophysiology of chronic fatigue syndrome. *Ciba Foundation Symposium, 173,* 176–192.

Lundgren, M., Persson, U., Larsson, P., Magnusson, C. I. E., Smith, L., Hammarstrom, L., & Severinson, E. (1989). Interleukin 4 induces synthesis of IgE and IgG4 in human B cells. *European Journal of Immunology, 19,* 1311–1315.

Lusso, P., Salahuddin, S. Z., Ablashi, D. V., Gallo, R.C., Di Marzo Veronese, F., & Markham, P. D. (1987). Diverse tropism of HBLV (human herpesvirus 6) (letter). *Lancet, 2,* 743–744.

MacDonald, K. L., Osterholm, M. T., LeDell, K. H., White, K. E., Schenck, C. H., Chao, C. C., Persing, D. H., Johnson, R. C., Baker, J. M., & Peterson, P. K. (1996). A case-control study to assess possible triggers and cofactors in chronic fatigue syndrome. *American Journal of Medicine,100,* 548–554.

Maeda, H., Kuwahara, H., Ichimura, Y., Ohtsuki, M., Kurakata, S., & Shiraishi, A. (1995). TGF-β enhances macrophage ability to produce IL-10 in mormal and tumor-bearing mice. *Journal of Immunology, 155,* 4926–4932.

Maeda, H., & Shiraishi, A. (1996). TGF-β contributes to the shift toward Th2-type responses through direct and IL-10-mediated pathways in tumor-bearing mice. *Journal of Immunology, 156,* 73–78.

McCluskey, D. R., & Riley, M. S. (1992). Chronic fatigue syndrome. *Comprehensive Therapy,18,* 13–16.

Modlin, R. L., & Nutman, T. B. (1993). Type 2 cytokines and negative immune regulation in human infections. *Current Opinion in Immunology, 5,* 511–517.

Moldofsky, H. (1993). Fibromyalgia, sleep disorder and chronic fatigue syndrome. *Ciba Foundation Symposium, 173,* 262–271. Discussion: 272–279.

Morris, A. G. (1988). Interferon. *Immunology, 1(1),* 43–45.

Morrison, L. J. A., Behan, W. H. M., & Nehan, P. O. (1991). Changes in natural killer cell phenotype in patients with post-viral fatigue syndrome. *Clinical and Experimental Immunology, 83,* 441–446.

Morriss, R., Sharpe, M., Sharpley, A. L., Cowen, P. J., Hawton, K., & Morris, J. (1993). Abnormalities of sleep in patients with the chronic fatigue syndrome. *British Medical Journal, 306*, 1161–1164.

Morte, S., Castilla, A., Civiera, M. P., Serrano, M., & Prietom, J. (1989). Production of interleukin-1 by peripheral blood mononuclear cells in patients with chronic fatigue syndrome. *Journal of Infectious Diseases, 159*, 362–367.

Mosmann, T. R., Chervinshi, H., Bond, M. W., Giedlin, M. A., & Coffman, R. L. T. (1986). Two types of murine helper T-cell clone. I. Definition according to profiles of lymphokine activities and secreted proteins. *Journal of Immunology,136*, 2348–2357.

Mosmann, T. R. (1991). Cytokines: is there biological meaning? *Current Opinion. in Immunology, 3*, 311–314.

Murdoch, J. C. (1988). Cell-mediated immunity in patients with myalgic encephalomyelitis syndrome. *New Zealand Medical Journal, 101*, 511–512.

Naor, D. (1992). Short analytical review. A different outlook at the phenotype-function relationships of T cell subpopulations. Fundamental and clinical implications. *Clinical Immunology and Immunopathology, 62*, 127–132.

O'Garra, A. (1989). Peptide regulatory factors. Interleukins and the immune system 1. *Lancet, 1*, 943–946.

O'Garra, A. (1989). Peptide regulatory factors. Interleukins and the immune system 2. *Lancet, 1*, 1003–1005.

Olson, G. B., Kanaan, M. N., Gersuk, G. M., Kelley, L. M., & Jones, J. F. (1986). Correlation between allergy and persistent Epstien-Barr virus infections in chronic active Epstein-Barr virus infected patients. *Journal of Allergy and Clinical Immunology,78*, 308–314.

Olson, G. B., Kanaan, M. N., Kelley, L. M., & Jones, J. F. (1986). Specific allergen-induced Epstein-Barr nuclear antigen-positive B cells from patients with chronic-active Epstein-Barr virus infections. *Journal of Allergy and Clinical Immunology, 78*, 315–320.

Opp, M. R., Smith, E. M., & Hughes, T. K. (1995). Interleukin-10 (cytokine synthesis inhibitory factor) acts in the central nervous system of rats to reduce sleep (short communication). *Journal of Neuroimmunology, 60*, 165–168.

Ortaldo, J. R., Mason, A. T., O'Shea, J. J., Smyth, M. J., Falk, L. A., Kennedy, I. C., Longo, D. L., & Ruscetti, F. W. (1991). Mechanistic studies of transforming growth factor-β inhibition of IL-2 dependent activation of CD3—large granular lymphocyte function. *Journal of Immunology, 146*, 3791–3798.

Oxelius, V. A., Hanson, L. A., Bjorkander, J., Hammarstrom, L., & Sjoholm, A. (1986). IgG3 deficiency, common in obstructive lung disease. *Monographs in Allergy, 20*, 106–115.

Patarca, R., Klimas, N. G., Lugtendorf, S., Antoni, M., & Fletcher, M. A. (1994). Dysregulated expression of tumor necrosis factor in chronic fatigue syndrome: interrelations with cellular sources and patterns of soluble immune mediator expression. *Clinical Infectious Diseases, 18(suppl 1)*, S147-s153.

Peterson, P. K., Sirr, S. A., Grammith, F. C., Schenck, C. H., Pheley, A. M., Hu, S., & Chao, C. C. (1994). Effects of mild exercise on cytokines and cerebral blood flow in chronic fatigue syndrome patients. *Clinical and Diagnostic Laboratory Immunology, 1(2)*, 222–226.

Prieto, J., Subir, M. L., Castilla, A., & Serrano, M. (1989). Naloxone reversible monocyte dysfunction in patients with chronic fatigue syndrome. *Scandinavian Journal of Immunology, 30*, 13–20.

Ristow, H. J. (1986). BSC-1 growth inhibitor/type β transforming growth factor is a strong inhibitor of thymocyte proliferation. *Proceedings of the National Academy of Sciences USA, 83*, 5531–5534.

Roberts, A. B., & Sporn, M. B. (1990). The transforming growth factor-β 5. In: M. B. Sporn & A. B. Roberts (Eds.),*Peptide Growth Factors and their Receptors* (pp. 421–472), Heidelberg: Springer-Verlag.

Romagnani, S. (1992). Human Th1 and Th2 subsets: regulation of differentiation and role in protection and immunopathology. *International Archives of Allergy Immunology, 98(4)*, 279–285.

Rook, A. H., Kehrl, J. H., Wakefield, L. M., Roberts, A. B., Sporn, M. B., Burlington, D. B., Lane, H. C., & Fauci, A. S. (1986). Effects of transforming growth factor-β on the function of natural killer cells: depressed cytolitic activity and blunting of interferon responsiveness. *Journal of Immunology, 136*, 3916–3920.

Rousset, F., Garcia, E., Defrance, T., Peronne, C., Vezzio, N., Hsu, D. H., Kastelein, R., Moore, K. W. , & Banchereau, J. (1992). Interleukin 10 is a potent growth and differentiation factor for activated human B lymphocytes. *Proceedings of the National Academy of Sciences USA. 89(5)*, 1890–1893.

Ruscetti, F., Vanesio, L., Ochoa, A., & Ontaldo, J. (1993). Pleiotropic effects of transforming growth factor-β on cells of the immune system. *Annals of New York Academy of Sciences, 685*, 488–500.

Schluesener, H., & Lider, O. (1989). Transforming growth factors β1 and β2: cytokines with identical immunosuppressive effects and a potential role in the regulation of autoimmune T cell function. *Journal of Neuroimmunology, 24*, 249–258.

Scott, P. (1993). Selective differentiation of CD4+ T helper cell subsets. *Current Opinion in Immunology, 5*, 391–397.

Sher, A., Gazzinelli, R. T., Oswald, I. P., Glerici, M., Kullberg, M., Pearce, E. J., Berzofsky, J. A., Mosmann, T, R., James, S. L., Morse, H. C., & Shearer, G. M. (1992). Role of T-cell-derived cytokines in the downregualtion of immune responses in parasitic and retroviral infection. *Immunological Review, 127*, 181–204.

Skavril, F. (1986). IgG subclasses in viral infections. *Monographs in Allergy, 19*, 134–143.

Snapper, C. M., & Paul, W. E. (1987). Interferon-γ and B cell stimulatory factor-1 reciprocally regulate Ig isotype production. *Science, 236*, 944–947.

Straus, S. E., Tosato, G., Armstrong, G., Lawley, T., Preble, O. T., Henle, W., Davey, R., Pearson, G., Epstein, J., & Brus, I. (1985). Persisting illness and fatigue in adults with evidence of Epstien-Barr virus infection. *Annals of Internal Medicine, 102*, 7–16.

Straus, S. E., Dale, J. K., Wright, R., & Metcalfe, D. D. (1988). Allergy and the chronic fatigue syndrome. *Journal of Allergy and Clinical Immunology, 81*, 791–795.

Sumaya, C. V. (1991). Serologic and virologic epidemiology of Epstien-Barr virus: relevance to chronic fatigue syndrome. *Review of Infectious Diseases,13(1)*, S19-S25.

Swanink, C. M. A., Vercoulen, J. H. M. M., Galama, J. M. D., Roos, M. T. L., Mcyaard, L., van der Ven-Jongekrijg, J., de Nijs, R., Bleijenberg, G., Fennis, J. F. M., Miedema, F., & van der Meer, J. W. M. (1996). Lymphocyte subsets, apoptosis, and cytokines in patients with chronic fatigue syndrome. *Journal of Infectious Diseases, 173*, 460–463.

Tosato, G., Straus, S., Henle, W., Pike, S, E., & Blaese, R. M. (1985). Characteristic T cell dysfunction in patients with chronic active Epstien-Barr virus infection (chronic infectious mononucleosis). *Journal of Immunology, 134*, 3082–3088.

Tovey, M. G., Content, J., Gresser, I., Gugenheim, J., Blanchard, B., Guymarho, J., Poupart, P., Gigon, M., Shaw, A., & Fiers, W. (1988). Genes for IFN-β-2 (IL-6), tumor necrosis factor, and IL-1 are expressed at high levels in the organs of normal individuals. *Journal of Immunology, 141*, 3106–3110.

Van Snick, J. (1990). Interleukin-6: an overview. *Annals of Review in Immunology, 8*, 253–278.

Wakefield, D., Lloyd, A., & Brockman, A. (1990). Immunoglobulin subclass abnormalities in patients with chronic fatigue syndrome. *Pediatric Infectious Diseases Journal, 9*, S50-S53.

Wakefield, D., Lloyd, A., Dwyer, J., Salahuddin, S. Z., & Ablashi, D. V. (1988). Human herpes-virus 6 and myalgic encephalomyelitis. *Lancet, 1*, 1059–1061.

Walh, S. M., Hunt, D. A., Wong, H. L., Dougherty, J., McCartney-Francis, N., Wahl, L. M., Ellingsworth, L., Schmidt, J. A., Hall, G., & Roberts, A. B. (1988). Transforming growth factor-β is a potent immunosuppressive agent that inhibits IL-1-dependent lymphocyte proliferation. *Journal of Immunology, 140*, 3026–3032.

Walh, S. M., McCartney-Francis, N. M., & Mergenhagen, S. E. (1989). Inflammatory and immunomodulatory roles of TGF-β. *Immunology Today, 10*, 258–261.

Wessely, S., & Powell, R. (1989). Fatigue syndromes: a comparison of chronic post-viral fatigue with neuromuscular and affective disorders. *Journal of Neurology, Neurosurgery and Psychiatry, 52,* 940–948.

Wong, G. C., & Clark, S. C. (1988). Multiple actions of interleukin 6 within a cytokine network. *Immunology Today, 9,* 137–139.

Wood, G. C., Bental, R. P., Gopfert, M., & Edwards, R. H. (1991). A comparative psychiatric assessment of patients with chronic fatigue syndrome and muscle disease. *Psychological Medicine, 21,* 619–628.

Yssel, H., Johnson, K. E., Schnieder, P. V., Wideman, J., Terr, A., Kastelein, R., & de Vries, J, E. (1992). T-cell activation-inducing epitopes of the house dust mite allergen Der p 1. Proliferation and lymphokine production patterns by Dr p 1-specific CD4+ T cell clones. *Journal of Immunology, 148,* 738–745.

8

CHRONIC FATIGUE SYNDROME: POSSIBLE INTEGRATION OF HORMONAL AND IMMUNOLOGICAL OBSERVATIONS

Abba J. Kastin, Richard D. Olson, J. Martin Martins,[*] Gayle A. Olson, James E. Zadina, and William A. Banks

VA Medical Center
Tulane University School of Medicine and
The University of New Orleans
New Orleans Louisiana 70146

1. INTRODUCTION

The editors of this book organized a meeting about an unusual syndrome—chronic fatigue syndrome (CFS). They also applied an unusual approach to the meeting by inviting us to give the "keynote conclusions". Although we have experience in both basic and clinical research ranging from peptide hormones to cytokines, we have no experience with CFS.

Initially we were skeptical about the wisdom of this approach and any contribution we could make to the diffi-

[*] JMM is a Visiting Endocrinologist from Curry Cabral Hospital, Lisbon, Portugal.

Chronic Fatigue Syndrome, edited by Yehuda and Mostofsky
Plenum Press, New York, 1997

culties associated with CFS. It is true that occasionally a new approach can shed light on an old problem, but our early interest was low. As our reading of the scientific literature progressed and after listening to the presentations at the meeting, related in the earlier chapters in this book, we began to change our view. We came to realize that we would be able to apply a fresh approach to the evaluation of the evidence accumulated in the field since 1990 and that we also might be able to offer a novel insight into the etiology of the problem.

It seemed to us that evidence was accumulating for two main causative factors in CFS. Each, by itself, could explain the fatigue and other symptoms. One involved decreased corticotropin (ACTH) releasing hormone (CRH) and the other involved increased activity of the cytokine interleukin 1 (IL-1α).

Rather than representing two opposing views, we realized that the observations about CRH and IL-1 fit together in a coherent pattern. To us the evidence clearly indicates that the decrease in CRH must have occurred before the increased activity of the cytokine and that they probably were causally related.

2. IS CFS A DISCRETE CONDITION?

2.1. Scientific vs. Popular Views

Shakespeare made a couple of statements that could be loosely applied to CFS by skeptics of its existence, reflecting the observation that although CFS may be a poorly documented syndrome, it nevertheless has attracted much public attention. He said: "The empty vessel makes the greatest sound" (Henry V. act IV. sc.4) and (out of context) "...full of sound and fury, signifying nothing" (Macbeth act V. sc.5).

The issue of whether there is an organic cause of CFS differs according to the type of publication in which it is discussed. In a paper published in the British Medical

Journal in 1994, MacLean and Wessely report the results of their search for papers on CFS published in the United Kingdom from 1980 (MacLeam & Wessely, 1994). They compared the views of the articles published in research journals with those in the medical trade press and popular press. Of the articles published in national newspapers and magazine, 69% favored organic causes for CFS. Of the articles in the professional press, 55% favored organic causes. However, of the articles in research journals, only 31% favored organic causes. The ratio of organic to inorganic causes of CFS increased with increasing distance from the medical community.

2.2. Problems with Laboratory Findings

Buchwald and Komaroff summarized five problems with many of the early studies of CFS (Buchwald & Komaroff, 1991).

    a. Patients may have been suffering from different illnesses in which fatigue is common. They felt that criteria for entry were not consistent among some studies, even those meeting fully the case definition of the Centers for Disease Control (CDC).

    b. Tests were often performed selectively.

    c. The time at which tests are performed during the course of CFS varied and sometimes were not even specified.

    d. There was no standardization among the laboratories performing the tests.

    e. Concurrent testing of matched healthy control subjects was usually lacking.

These authors (Buchwald & Komaroff, 1991) concluded that the abnormal laboratory tests reported in CFS can be diverse, conflicting, and modest in degree. They were most impressed by the immunological dysfunction and called for systematic, blinded studies including healthy control subjects.

2.3. Problems with Statistical Analyses

Because of the interdisciplinary nature of the study of chronic fatigue syndrome, articles published on this topic vary greatly in their use of statistical analyses. To help reduce further confusion in this field, it is recommended that all future studies using inferential statistical procedures should include appropriate values for power, statistical significance, and effects size. Examination of all three of these values will lead to a better understanding of the results of the study. A discussion of these topics is included in the Appendix (section 11.).

2.4. Epidemiology

A specific viral etiology for CFS has not been established. Epidemics of CFS would be consistent with such a cause. One author felt that the recent increase in cases does suggest that a predominant agent is involved (Levy, 1994). However, as Fukuda clearly points out elsewhere in this book, CFS is sporadic, not epidemic, in nature. Sudden increased awareness and "popularity" of a syndrome also could convey the false impression of an epidemic.

2.5. Psychiatric Illness

The role of depression in CFS is discussed earlier in this volume. In some studies showing an increased incidence of mental depression in patients with CFS, the cases tended not to meet the CDC criteria for CFS (Deluca, Johnson, & Natelson, 1994). Memory deficits were found to be of a different pattern than those in depressed patients (Sandman, Barron, Nackoul, Goldstein, & Fidler, 1993). There even has been a report of better performance on tests of concentration, attention, and abstraction in CFS than in age-matched normal controls, emphasizing the discrepancy between subjective complaints of cognitive impairment and objective performance (Altay et al., 1990).

Preexistence of depression is difficult to determine in CFS, particularly because the original (Holmes et al.,

1988) CDC criteria for CFS excluded cases with previously diagnosed mental illness such as endogenous depression. The newer criteria of the CDC exclude major psychotic depression but not less severe forms of depression since it is felt that such psychiatric conditions are highly prevalent in persons with CFS (Fukuda et al., 1994).

Certainly, chronic fatigue could result in symptoms of depression and depression could result in symptoms of chronic fatigue. One study attempted to control for the chronicity of CFS and its higher ratio of females by using a control group of patients with rheumatoid arthritis (Katon, Buchwald, Simon, Russo, & Mease, 1991). Higher levels of psychiatric illness were found in the patients with CFS than in the patients with rheumatoid arthritis.

Perhaps more meaningful was the higher prevalence of lifetime major depression in CFS, being 85.7% vs. 48.4% in controls in one study (Katon, Buchwald, Simon, Russo, & Mease, 1991) and 78% vs. 22% in another study (Gold et al., 1990). However, this was not a universal finding (Hickie, Lloyd, Wakefield, & Parker, 1990). Extraordinarily high rates of current and lifetime psychiatric disorders also were found in the patients with CFS who had the highest number of medically unexplained physical symptoms (Katon & Russo, 1992). Another group of investigators, making use of the important statistical tool of power analysis emphasized elsewhere in this article, found that the strongest independent predictors of postinfectious fatigue were the fatigue and psychological distress existing before onset of the infection (Wessely et al., 1995). An NIH study found high rates (75%) of psychiatric illness in patients with CFS and concluded that "the high lifetime prevalence of psychiatric disorders in our patients, as well as the increased likelihood of psychiatric illness predating the chronic fatigue, suggests that psychiatric factors contribute to the pathogenesis of the chronic fatigue syndrome" (Kruesi, Dale, & Straus, 1989).

Abbey and Garfinkel argue that "the majority of [CFS] sufferers are experiencing primary psychiatric disorders or psychophysiological reactions and that the disorder is often a culturally sanctioned form of illness behavior" (Abbey & Garfinkel, 1991). The controversial place held by psychiatric illness in CFS is illustrated by the critical letters published a year later in response to this article (Am. J. Psychiatry 149: 1753–1757, 1992). In addition, as will be seen later in this article, basal concentrations of cortisol in the plasma and responses of prolactin to serotonergic stimulation differ in CFS and depression; even this, however, does not preclude an early contributory role for depression.

3. CONFUSING LABORATORY FINDINGS REPORTED IN THE '90S FOR CFS

3.1. Lymphocyte Phenotypes

Realizing that no clear picture of immunologic abnormalities existed in the CFS literature taken as a whole, we hoped that analysis of only the more recent literature from the '90s might yield more consistent results. By this time, the CDC criteria would have been in place and newer laboratory techniques available. As can be seen in Tables 1 and 2, we were disappointed. Much overlap between reports of normal and abnormal findings exists.

It did seem, however, as if some findings were reported more often than others. Altered CD8 cells were among these (Buchwald et al., 1992; Klimas, Salvato, Morgan, & Fletcher, 1990; Landay, Jessop, Lennette, & Levy, 1991; Levy, Landay, Jessop, & Lennette, 1993) in some, but not all studies (Chao et al., 1991), as were some (Straus, Fritz, Dale, Gould, & Strober, 1993; Buchwald et al., 1992) but not all (Levy, Landay, Jessop, & Lennette, 1993; Chao et al., 1991) studies of CD4 T cells. This may depend upon the subset analyzed (Klimas, Salvato, Morgan, & Fletcher, 1990). Another frequently reported abnormality is reduction in natural killer (NK) cells (Klimas, Salvato, Morgan, & Fletcher, 1990; Gupta & Vayuvegula,

Table 1. Abnormal lymphocyte phenotypes reported in 90's for CFS

T cell subsets	T cell activation
↓CD4	↑CD8 HLA-DR
↓CD4/CD8	↑CD8 IL
↓CD45RA	↑CD8 11b
↑CD45RO	↓CD8 11b-
↓CD4 CD45RA	↑CD8 CD38
↑CD8	NK cells
↑CD8 CD45RO	↓Cytotoxicity
↑CD8 12	↑CD56
↑CD2 CDw26	Cell adhesion
B cell subsets	↑CD45RO CD29
↑CD20	↑CD45RO CD54
↑CD5 CD20	↑CD45RO CD58
↑CD21	

Table 2. Normal lymphocyte phenotypes reported in 90's for CFS

Total t cells	Cell adhesion markers
CD3	CD44
CD5	CD54
T cell subsets	NK cells
CD4	CD16
CD25	CD57
CD29	CD4 CD57
CD8	CD8 CD56
CD4/CD8	CD16 CD56
CD4 CD5	Macrophages
CD4 CD45RO	CD11
CD4 CD45RA	CD11A CD18
CD45RA CD45RO	CD15
B cell subsets	Cell adhesion
CD20	CD4 CD29
CD20 CD5	CD4 CD11a
CD20 CD23	CD4 CD54
CD20 CD45RO	CD4 CD58
T cell activation	CD45RA CD29
CD4 IL2R	CD45RA CD11a
CD8 IL2R	CD45RA CD54
CD4 HLA-DR	CD45RA CD58
CD8 CD11b	CD45RO CD11a
CD8 CD38	

1991), but this was not a uniform finding (Landay, Jessop, Lennette, & Levy, 1991; Levy, Landay, Jessop, & Lennette, 1993; Rasmussen et al., 1994). In another context, our laboratory had difficulty reproducing frequently reported findings with NK cells (Kastin, Seligson, Strimas, & Chi, 1991). This may reflect an inherent variability in determination of NK cell activity that may contribute to the differing results in studies dependent upon such measurements such as some of those of CFS.

Although many of the results with lymphocyte phenotypes are consistent with chronic stimulation of the immune system, they are relatively nonspecific and fail to represent a consistently characteristic or diagnostic immunological test for the diagnosis of CFS.

3.2. Miscellaneous Laboratory Findings

In an attempt to obtain a better understanding of CFS as well as a characteristic or diagnostic test, several additional substances were measured (Gupta & Vayuvegula, 1991; Rasmussen et al., 1994; Lloyd, Hickie, Brockman, Dwyer, & Wakefield, 1991). In general, these were all reported as normal, as summarized in Table 3.

Table 3. Normal misc. lab. findings
reported in '90s for CFS

WBC
Monocytes
Neoptyrin (+CSF)
IgM
IgG (t,1,2,3,4)
IgA
ANA
Anti-ssDNA Ab
Anti-smooth & striated muscle Ab
Anti-RNP Ab
Anti-mitochondrial Ab
Anti-cardiolipin Ab
Anti-thyroid peroxidase Ab

4. VIRAL STUDIES

Most of the laboratory tests listed in Tables 1–3 are usually associated with changes occurring after a viral illness. Indeed, for a long time CFS was called chronic Epstein-Barr virus syndrome and Coxsackie viruses were frequently implicated.

A large number of viruses have been evaluated since the '90s (Landay, Jessop, Lennette, & Levy, 1991; Levy, Landay, Jessop, & Lennette, 1993; Buchwald et al., 1992; Miller et al., 1991; Khan et al., 1993; Gow et al., 1992; De-Freitas et al., 1991; Heneine et al., 1994; Folks et al., 1993). They are listed in Table 4. In one of the few areas of agreement among workers in the field, it is now acknowledged that no one virus can be implicated as the causative agent for CFS, although some positive findings continue to be reported. This, as well as other features of CFS, are well summarized elsewhere (Mawle, Reyes, & Schmid, 1994).

Table 4. Normal viral findings reported in '90s for CFS

EBV (EA & EBNA)
Coxsackie B
CMV
SPUMA retroviruses
Rubeola
Adenovirus 2
Papovavirus (BK)
HTLV-I,II
HIV- 1,2
HSV
HHV-6
2 (HTLV-II) *gag*
Enterovirus
Bovine leukemia virus
Feline leukemia virus
Gibbon ape leukemia virus
Simian t-lymphotropic virus
Simian retroviruses 1,2, & 3

Table 5. Abnormal viral findings
reported in '90s for CFS

↑HHV-6
↑EBV
↑SPUMA retroviruses
↑HTLV
↑2 (HTLV-II) *gag*

5. TREATMENT

As might be expected for a disease with no proven
cause, treatment is not very successful. These therapies
have been summarized elsewhere (Wilson, Hickie, Lloyd, &
Wakefield, 1994; Goodnick & Sandoval, 1993). Perhaps the
most complete discussion, including cognitive behavior
therapy, is provided by Fukuda and

Gantz (Fukuda & Gantz, 1995). The drugs tried in
CFS are summarized in Table 6.

Table 6. Some of the types of drugs tried in Rx of CFS

Antibacterial (e.g., doxycycline)
Antidepressants
TCA
SSRA
RIMA
MAOI
Antifungals (e.g., ketoconazole)
Anti-inflammatory agents
Antiviral (e.g., acyclovir)
ß-Adrenergic receptor antagonists (e.g., atenolol)
Calcium-channel blockers (e.g., nifedipine)
Essential fatty acids
H_2 receptor antagonists
Immune modifiers (e.g., Ampligen, transfer factor, IFN-α, kutapressin, immunoglobulin, and dialyzable leukocyte extract)
Opiate antagonists (e.g., naltrexone)
Psychoactive agents (e.g., benzodiazepines)
Stimulants (e.g., amphetamines)
Vitamins and minerals (e.g., Mg)

6. CRH DEFICIENCY

In contrast to the earlier quotations from Shakespeare that could be applied to a skeptical interpretation of the reality of CFS, an even earlier quotation could be loosely applied as supporting the existence of CFS. Plautus (254–184 BC) said "There is no smoke without fire". Similarly, J. Lyly (1554–1606) said: "There can be no great smoke arise, but there must be some fire". We believe that the relative deficiency in CRH in CFS might represent the spark for that possible fire.

6.1. In CFS

Perhaps the most prominent symptom of adrenal insufficiency is fatigue. Adrenal insufficiency arises at one of three anatomic sites:

    a. adrenals (Addison's disease), resulting in a deficiency of cortisol and other adrenal hormones
    b. pituitary, resulting in a deficiency of ACTH
    c. hypothalamus, resulting in a deficiency of CRH.

A deficiency at a higher site (e.g., hypothalamus) results in a deficiency at a lower (e.g., pituitary and adrenal) site.

Demitrack et al. (Demitrack et al., 1991) performed a thorough examination of the hypothalamic-pituitary-adrenal (HPA) axis in 30 patients with CFS and compared the results with those from 72 normal volunteers. The patients with CFS showed reduced concentrations of cortisol and increased concentrations of ACTH in the evening (unfortunately no results are reported for the morning), decreased excretion of free cortisol in 24 hour samples of urine, and increased sensitivity of the adrenals to ACTH associated with a diminished maximal response. Furthermore, compared with controls, the patients with CFS showed an attenuated net integrated pituitary release of ACTH in response to CRH. Concentrations of CRH in the cerebrospinal fluid (CSF) were no different from controls

(Demitrack et al., 1991), a finding difficult to interpret because of the specific transport system for CRH out of, but not into, the brain (Martins, Kastin, & Banks, 1996).

If the adrenals were the main location of the defect in the HPA, as could be inferred from the evening values, they probably would not have shown an enhanced response to the administration of ACTH. Moreover, primary adrenal insufficiency would not readily explain the blunted response of the pituitary to CRH.

If the pituitary were the main location of the defect, the concentrations of ACTH should not have been increased at any time. The blunted response of the pituitary to CRH is compatible with a chronic decrease of stimulation associated with diminished CRH. As the authors conclude (Demitrack et al., 1991), this indicates that the hypothalamus, the source of CRH, is the main site of the defect in the HPA even though some of the results are compatible with a relative primary adrenal defect. In this regard, the increasing recognition of the relatively high incidence of mild forms of late-onset congenital adrenal hyperplasia suggests another group to be compared with CFS. An earlier study compared 25 patients with fatigue with 25 normal subjects matched for age and sex (Poteliakhoff, 1981). They found decreased concentrations of cortisol in the plasma in both acute and chronic fatigue. Studies such as this have convinced Jefferies (Jefferies, 1994) that mild adrenocortical deficiency exists in CFS. A later study found that basal cortisol concentrations in the blood of patients with CFS tended to be lower than in healthy controls and were much lower than in depressed patients (Cleare et al., 1995).

6.2. In Stress

Chronic or repeated complex stress can be characterized by a loss of diurnal rhythm with relatively normal circulating concentrations of ACTH and glucocorticoids (Harbuz & Lightman, 1992). In contrast to the study mentioned above where adrenal hypofunction was found associated with both acute and chronic fatigue (Poteliakhoff, 1981), hypothalamic CRH levels probably are different in these two conditions. In acute stress, concentrations of CRH generally are increased, whereas in chronic stress they can be decreased (Harbuz & Lightman, 1992; Moldow, Kastin, Graf, & Fischman, 1987; Flier & Underhill, 1995; Swain, Patchev, Vergalla, Chrousos, & Jones, 1993; Dallman, 1993; De Goeij, Binnekade, & Tilders, 1992).

Swain et al. (Swain, Patchev, Vergalla, Chrousos, & Jones, 1993) examined surgically operated rats exposed to ether vapor. They found decreased ACTH responses to CRH accompanied by decreased hypothalamic content of CRH as well as decreased expression of CRH MRNA in the paraventricular nucleus (PVN) of the hypothalamus. This was accompanied by a decreased release of CRH from hypothalamic explants of these rats.

A similar apparently paradoxical fall in CRH MRNA in the PVN was found by another group in a different animal model involving chronic inflammatory stress (Harbuz et al., 1992). This decline in CRH message was accompanied by a corresponding decrease in the release of CRH into the hypophyseal portal blood. The authors point out that in contrast to acute stress, in chronic stress there is habituation or adaptation of the increased activity of the HPA axis to the stressful stimulus, resulting in an attenuated response.

Although decreased concentrations of CRH in chronic stress might be associated with its increased release, another study also showed that this was caused by a temporal suppression of the production of CRH in the PVN (De Goeij, Binnekade, & Tilders, 1992). This study used repeated insulin-induced hypoglycemia as its stress whereas another study (Chappell et al., 1986) in which decreased concentrations of CRH were found used a 13-day course of several unpredictable stressors. The results of these investigations show that several types of chronic stress can result in decreased CRH synthesis and release in animals, resembling the findings in CFS.

It must be cautioned that stress is a heterogeneous condition and still poorly understood. The response to stress is influenced by many variables ranging from neonatal events (Meaney et al., 1991; Reul et al., 1994) to genetic predisposition (Aubry et al., 1995; Zhukov, 1993). Nevertheless, this does not mean that consideration of stress should be ignored in conditions like CFS.

Thus, in contrast to some popular views, chronic stress can result in some circumstances in impaired function of the HPA. If a deficiency of CRH plays a role in CFS, then it is possible that chronic stress could be a major causative factor. Stress often precedes the onset of CFS (Holmes et al., 1988).

6.3. In Females

Adrenal insufficiency, like CFS, is more common in females. Since the vast majority of cases of adrenal insufficiency result from autoimmune disease at the primary site of the adrenals, it is not known whether tertiary adrenal insufficiency at the hypothalamic level also is more common in females.

There is a strain of rats (Lewis) that is more susceptible to inflammatory and autoimmune disease. They show an impaired response of their HPA axis in response to stress. As was seen in patients with CFS (Demitrack et al., 1991), these rats also show a diminished ACTH response to CRH. This defect is more common in female rats (Spinedi et al., 1994). They also show markedly impaired ACTH release in response to rhIL-1α and a serotonin agonist (Sternberg et al., 1989).

Autoimmune disease, in general, is more common in women. If this phenomenon is related to levels of estrogen, then the increased use of this steroid in postmenopausal females might be correlated with an increased incidence of autoimmune disease in this older group, a possible correlation that could be tested.

7. IL-1α INCREASE

7.1. In CFS

Now that it is possible to measure IL-1α by immunoassay, this was done in the '90s by two groups. The one in Stockholm used an enzyme-linked immunosorbent assay (ELISA) and the one in Miami used radioimmunoassay (RIA) in the blood of patients meeting the CDC criteria for CFS. In each study, increased concentrations of IL-1α were found (Linde et al., 1992; Patarca, Klimas, Lugtendorf, Antoni, & Fletcher, 1994; Patarca, Fletcher, & Klimas, 1993). Neither group found an accompanying increase in the serum concentrations of IL-1β, which agrees with other studies in which IL-1β but not IL-1α were measured (Straus, Dale, Peter, & Dinarello, 1989; Lloyd, Gandevia, Brockman, Hales, & Wakefield, 1994; Lloyd, Hickie, Brockman, Dwyer, & Wakefield, 1991).

In the Swedish study, 74.3% of the 35 patients with CFS were women and in the Miami study 90.8% of the patients were women. These were compared with 20 and 53 control subjects respectively, both groups comprised of blood donors. Although increased concentrations of IL-1α only occurred in a relatively small percent of the patients with CFS, in at least one of the studies the top quartile in terms of disability had the highest level of IL-1 (Patarca, Fletcher, & Klimas, 1993). It is possible that this number would be higher at different times during the course of the disease. In a section of JAMA called "Medical News & Perspectives", Cotton mentions one study in which more than two thirds of all CFS patients had markedly elevated concentrations of IL-1 and IL-2 and another, at Miami, in which 42% of patients had elevated concentrations of IL-1α (Cotton, 1991).

Great care was taken in the immunoassays in these two studies. For the ELISA, samples from the healthy controls were examined in parallel with those from CFS to exclude the possibility that cytokines were released during storage or preparation of the blood samples (Linde et al.,

1992). To verify the sensitivity of the assay, it was checked for the increases expected during bacterial infections; none of the controls had increased concentrations. The antibodies were elicited against rhDNA-produced IL-1α. Specificity was tested with 10,000-fold excess of IL-1ß and IgG fractions from nonimmunized rabbits run in parallel. For the RIA, quality controls with recombinant and natural cytokines were performed, and variability was <10% (Patarca, Klimas, Lugtendorf, Antoni, & Fletcher, 1994).

The Swedish study (Linde et al., 1992) contained an additional group of controls composed of patients with Epstein-Barr virus infection considered to have infectious mononucleosis. Although they also had increased concentrations of IL-1α in their serum acutely (not more than 7 days after onset), 6 months later only the group with CFS maintained significantly increased concentrations. Moreover, the group with CFS lacked most of the markers for lymphocyte activation that were found in the patients with infectious mononucleosis.

In the Miami study (Patarca, Klimas, Lugtendorf, Antoni, & Fletcher, 1994), reverse transcriptase-coupled polymerase chain reaction revealed no messenger RNA for IL-1α in peripheral blood mononuclear cells or granulocytes of several patients with CFS and increased IL-1α. This implies that the IL-1α in CFS is probably derived from a source other than peripheral blood cells. Another study was reported in the '90s using the older *in vitro* method in LPS/PHA-stimulated mononuclear cells incubated for 18 hours at 37°C (Rasmussen et al., 1994). The stimulated values, several hundred times higher than normal concentrations in blood, were not significantly different in samples from patients with CFS and controls.

Most patients with CFS have disorders of sleep that can contribute to the fatigue (Morris et al., 1993). Earlier in this book, and elsewhere (Moldofsky, 1995), Moldofsky has ably summarized the evidence for a link between IL-1α and the sleep-wake disturbances characteristic of CFS. He points out that serotonin also can promote slow wave sleep.

7.2. In Stimulating the HPA Axis

IL-1α activates the HPA axis by acting primarily at the hypothalamic level (Suda et al., 1990). It does so by stimulating gene expression of CRH with accompanying release of CRH and, secondarily, ACTH. Most of the early studies showing potent stimulation of the HPA axis by IL-1 used IL-1ß and are well summarized elsewhere (Wick, Hu, Schwarz, & Kroemer, 1993), but IL-1α has been shown to be as effective as IL-1ß (Imura, Fukata, & Mori, 1991; Suda et al., 1990).

7.3. Can IL-1 Cross the Blood Brain Barrier (BBB)?

Like the popular misconceptions that at one time plagued the peptide field, it has been assumed by some investigators that cytokines are too large to cross the BBB. This is not true.

IL-1α is transported across the BBB by a saturable system so that it has direct access to cortical (including hypothalamic) brain and spinal cord cells (Banks, Kastin, & Gutierrez, 1993; Banks, Kastin, & Ehrensing, 1994) without disrupting the BBB (Banks & Kastin, 1992). This transport system is shared with IL-1ß (Banks, Ortiz, Plotkin, & Kastin, 1991) but not with IL-2 (Waguespack, Banks, & Kastin, 1994), TNF-α (Barrera, Banks, Fasold, & Kastin, 1991), IL-6 (Banks, Kastin, & Gutierrez, 1994), or the MIPs (Banks & Kastin, 1996). IL-1α alone is selectively transported from the blood into the posterior division of the septum of the mouse brain (Maness, Banks, Zadina, & Kastin, 1995) and can be blocked by preincubation with its soluble receptor (Banks, Plotkin, & Kastin, 1995).

8. SEROTONIN INCREASE

8.1. In CFS

Demitrack et al. (Demitrack et al., 1992) found that basal plasma levels of 5-hydroxyindoleacetic acid (5-HIAA) were significantly increased in 19 patients (13 women) meeting the CDC criteria for CFS as compared with 17 normal subjects. Serotonin (5-hydroxytrptamine: 5-HT), found in high concentrations in the hypothalamus, is converted by the monoamine oxidase (MAO) enzyme both pre- and postsynaptically to its principal inactive metabolite 5-HIAA. In the CSF, these concentrations did not differ between the groups.

Using an indirect measure of serotonin receptors, Bakheit et al. (Bakheit, Behan, Dinan, Gray, & O'Keane, 1992) found evidence for upregulation of hypothalamic serotonin receptors in 15 patients with CFS as compared with 13 age- and sex-matched healthy subjects and 13 patients with primary depression. They showed this by measuring prolactin release in response to buspirone, a 5-HT$_{1A}$ receptor agonist that also may have other properties, including those on the release of prolactin, which may confound the results. Similarly increased prolactin release in CFS also was found in response to fenfluramine in patients with CFS as compared with controls matched for age, weight, sex, and stage of menstrual cycle (Cleare et al., 1995).

8.2. On HPA

Serotonin directly stimulates the secretion of CRH from the hypothalamus (Calogero, Gallucci, Gold, & Chrousos, 1988; Hu, Lightman, & Tannahill, 1992; Hillhouse & Milton, 1989). Among the multiple serotonin receptors in brain, the 5-HT$_{1A}$ receptor is one that mediates activation both of the HPA and prolactin release (Bagdy & Makara, 1994). Differential activity of the various serotonin receptors on pituitary hormones and CRH has been shown, although some, like 5-HT$_3$ receptors, are not involved in the serotonergic stimulation of ACTH release (Levy, Quan, Rittenhouse, & Van de Kar, 1993; Bagdy & Makara, 1994; Calogero et al., 1989).

The PVN of the hypothalamus is involved in the 5-HT$_{1A}$ induced release of ACTH, but not prolactin, after neural stimulation (Bagdy & Makara, 1994; Feldman, Conforti, & Melamed, 1987). 5-HT$_{1A}$ binding sites in the hippocampus and cortex are also affected by adrenalectomy and administration of corticosterone (the main glucocorticoid of the rat) (Mendelson & McEwen, 1992).

9. VASOPRESSIN DEFICIENCY

The PVN also is the site of production of arginine vasopressin (AVP). A single study of 9 patients with CFS showed lower baseline concentrations of AVP than in the 8 healthy controls (Bakheit, Behan, Watson, & Morton, 1993). In contrast to the controls, patients with CFS did not show a close correlation between serum osmolality and plasma AVP concentrations in response to a water load, indicating a deficient responsiveness of the release of AVP.

AVP, like CRH, stimulates the pituitary gland to secrete ACTH. This action appears to occur through a separate pathway, resulting in a synergistic action. It is conceivable that a disorder affecting CRH also could affect AVP.

10. CRH DECREASE AND IL-1α INCREASE: WHICH CAME FIRST?

This resembles the proverbial question of the chicken and the egg, except that this time there is evidence to indicate which did come first.

10.1. Is It the IL-1α?

No.

More investigations of immune disorders in CFS have been published than of hormonal disorders. If medical decisions were judged by the number or weight of the published studies, then we would still be thinking that peptic ulcers were caused by emotional stress rather than by bacteria. The situation is similar with other scientific issues. By this reasoning, immune matters would be primary for CFS.

However, as we showed in section 7.2 of this invited chapter, IL-1 stimulates the release of CRH. Therefore, if the primary problem in CFS involved increased levels of IL-1, then the levels of CRH, ACTH, and cortisol would be increased, which they were not.

10.2. Is It the CRH?

Yes.

10.2.1. Can It Explain the Increased IL-1α? Yes. If the primary problem in CFS involved decreased concentrations of CRH, then the observed increase in the concentrations of IL-1 would be expected on the basis of classic negative feedback. Conversely, glucocorticoids inhibit IL-1 production as well as some peripheral actions (Wick, Hu, Schwarz, & Kroemer, 1993). Thus, decreased concentrations of CRH would be expected to lead to increased concentrations of IL-1. To remain low, the defect at the level of CRH would be severe.

10.2.2. Does It Explain the Increased Serotonin? Yes. By the same type of negative feedback just mentioned, serotonin activity should be increased by decreased concentrations of CRH. Both dexamethasone and aldosterone reduce serotonin-activated release of CRH (Hu, Lightman, & Tannahill, 1992). This also might explain the findings that the stresses of chronic restraint (Adell, Garcia-Marquez, Armario, & Gelpi, 1988) and exercise to fatigue (Blomstrand, Perrett, Parry-Billings, & Newsholme, 1989) increase the concentrations of serotonin and its metabolite 5-HIAA in the hypothalamus. These results together with indirect findings involving ingestion by marathon runners of tryptophan, the precursor of serotonin, have led to the hypothesis that increased serotonin in the brain may play a causative role in fatigue (Newsholme, Blomstrand, Hassmen, & Ekblom, 1991).

10.2.3. Does It Explain the Fatigue? Yes. Decreased concentrations of cortisol and increased concentrations of IL-1α and possibly serotonin can explain the fatigue of CFS.

10.2.4. Is This the Final Answer? Hardly. Although even some investigators who performed the key studies showing decreased CRH remain doubtful that CFS represents a discrete disease with a singular cause (Demitrack, 1994), they did not consider that decreased CRH can explain the increased IL-1α as well as other findings (e.g. increased serotonin) characteristic of CFS. Our main contribution, if any, is to suggest that if CRH and IL-1 are etiological factors in CFS, then the decrease in CRH probably occurs before the increase in IL-1, or even serotonin, although simultaneous unexplained actions on each are conceivable.

This may be considered too novel a concept, but it also has implications extending back to some of the original thinking about stress and CFS. Based on animal studies described elsewhere in this chapter (section 6.2), there is evidence that chronic stress can decrease CRH.

11. APPENDIX: STATISTICAL ANALYSES

Traditionally, statistical analysis has focused on determination of the probabilistic significance of the inferential test. First, a null hypothesis is established that typically states there is no difference between the means of the populations from which the test samples have been drawn. Then the means of the test samples are compared with an inferential test such as the analysis of variance (ANOVA). When the difference between treatment means is substantial enough to produce a test value (e.g., ANOVA produces an *F* value) so large that it might be expected less than 5% of the time by chance, it is generally concluded that the

null hypothesis should be rejected and that the groups being tested are probably different; i.e., the samples have
been drawn from different populations.

Unfortunately, because we are making a probabilistic
judgement, sometimes we make mistakes. For example,
part of the time when the null hypothesis is rejected because the test value is so large, it is not because the populations from which the samples were drawn were different
but only because random sampling led to samples drawn
from different extreme values of an identical population.
Accordingly, when this occurs, the erroneous conclusion is
drawn that a real difference existed and that finding is
published prematurely.

This statistical rarity, therefore, could lead to different
investigators obtaining different results when trying to replicate the original findings and thereby generate conflicts
in the literature. Although 95% of the time in this example
statistical significance would not be obtained, 5% of the
time it would; thus whereas this error is relatively rare, a
5% error rate is still frequent enough to cause considerable problems in the literature.

The easiest solution to this problem is to always replicate your findings, especially when they are novel or controversial. Replication of the finding several times provides
a strong argument for the validity of the results, but it is
time-consuming and costly.

A more sophisticated statistical solution is to add the
calculations of effect size and power to all of the analyses
involving statistical significance. Effect size is the proportion of the experimental variance that can be explained by
treatment, as opposed to the unexplained variance caused
by all other factors.

There are many measures of effect size, but most statistical packages routinely generate R^2 and partial eta
squared. The squared multiple correlation coefficient, R^2,
is usually provided for the total model effect, which is the
sum of all individual treatment effects, and is a ratio of
the variance that can be attributed to the sum of all treatment groups divided by the total variance. Partial eta

squared, however, is provided separately for each treatment effect in the model. It is a ratio of the variance explained by a given treatment effect divided by the sum of that same variance plus the unexplained variance; the denominator does not contain the variance explained by the other treatment effects. The importance of these measures is that they are relatively independent of sample size and give a more direct measure of the meaning of the numerical results, with the higher the value obtained for effect size, the better.

Much published research seems to yield partial eta squared values between 0.10 and 0.40, with values higher than that being increasingly more difficult to obtain. Whereas partial eta squared is the preferred measure of effect size for a given treatment, it is by necessity a relative measure and will be influenced by the number of variables in the design of the study and the amount of variance attributed to each of them. Thus, within a given study, the immediate value of partial eta squared is to provide a direct comparison of the relative importance of the variables being studied.

What is desirable is consistency between the probabilistic results of statistical significance and the analysis of effect size. Usually the results correlate nicely and the investigator reaches the correct statistical decision. In general, failure to obtain statistical significance is typically because the effect size is too small. However, statistical significance is usually obtained when the effect size is substantial.

Statistical significance may be thought of as the product of sample size multiplied by effect size, and this is what sometimes causes problems. Studies that explain very little variance and, therefore, have small partial eta squared values may still be misleadingly significant if the sample size is large. Conversely, studies that explain much of the variance but use very small sample sizes may not yield statistical significance, which can be an equally misleading problem for a worthwhile study. If only one statistic is used to analyze the data, some measure of effect size could actually be more meaningful than a significance level from an inferential test.

The problem, therefore, becomes the difficulty in determination of what is the correct sample size for the experiment being planned. This answer may be calculated by power analysis, the third component of contemporary statistical analysis. Before the beginning of the study, power analysis enables the investigator to take into account the hypothesized differences between treatment groups and the amount of variability expected so as to determine a probability value for power for a range of potential sample sizes. As sample size increases and the other values stay the same, power increases. Technically, power is the probability of rejecting the null hypothesis when it is false; i.e., making a correct decision. Practically, it is the probability of being able to replicate your findings.

Although the desired value of power is not as universally agreed upon as the value of 0.05 for determination of statistical significance, the field is moving toward a value of 0.80. The power must be high enough that the experiment is likely to be replicated, but there is no need to waste time or expense to raise the power to .90 or .95, which would require a tremendous increase in sample size. Power planning tables enable the determination of sample size before data are collected, so as to yield the value of power that is desired.

This produces a situation in which all research should start with power planning and determine a sample size that generates a value of power close to 0.80. Then, when that sample size is multiplied by the obtained effect size value, statistical significance will be more likely to lead to correct interpretations of data and produce fewer conflicts in the literature.

As evidence of the growing realization that these three measures must be evaluated jointly, the American Psychological Association recently required that all three values be included in articles submitted for publication in its journals, and others will soon be following this policy. Accordingly, at this time, it would be helpful if all future publications using inferential statistical tests would include power, statistical significance, and effect size. This would be particularly helpful in the study of a controversial disorder like CFS.

REFERENCES

Abbey, S.E. & Garfinkel, P.E. (1991). Neurasthenia and chronic fatigue syndrome: the role of culture in the making of a diagnosis. *American Journal of Psychiatry, 148,* 1638–1646.

Adell, A., Garcia-Marquez, C., Armario, A., & Gelpi, E. (1988). Chronic stress increases serotonin and noradrenaline in rat brain and sensitizes their responses to a further acute stress. *Journal of Neurochemistry, 50,* 1678–1681.

Altay, H.T., Toner, B.B., Brooker, H., Abbey, S.E., Salit, I.E., & Garfinkel, P.E. (1990). The neuropsychological dimensions of postinfectious neuromy asthenia (chronic fatigue syndrome): a preliminary report. *International Journal of Psychiatry in Medicine, 20,* 141–149.

Aubry, J.-M., Bartanusz, V., Driscoll, P., Schulz, P., Steimer, T., & Kiss, J.Z. (1995). Corticotropin-releasing factor and vasorpessin mRNA levels in roman high- and low-avoidance rats: response to open-field exposure. *Neuroendocrinology, 61,* 89–97.

Bagdy, G. & Makara, G.B. (1994). Hypothalamic paraventricular nucleus lesions differentially affect serotonin-1A (5-HT$_{1A}$) and 5-HT$_2$ receptor agonist-induced oxytocin, prolactin, and corticosterone responses. *Endocrinology, 134,* 1127–1131.

Bakheit, A.M.O., Behan, P.O., Dinan, T.G., Gray, C.E., & O'Keane, V. (1992). Possible upregulation of hypothalamic 5-hydroxytryptamine receptors in patients with postviral fatigue syndrome. *British Medical Journal, 304,* 1010–1012.

Bakheit, A.M.O., Behan, P.O., Watson, W.S., & Morton, J.J. (1993). Abnormal arginine-vasopressin secretion and water metabolism in patients with postviral fatigue syndrome. *ACTA Neurologica Scandinavica, 87(3),* 234–238.

Banks, W.A & Kastin, A.J. (1992). The interleukins-1α, -1β, and -2 do not acutely disrupt the murine blood-brain barrier. *International Journal of Immunopharmacology, 14,* 629–636.

Banks, W.A & Kastin, A.J. (1996). Reversible association of the cytokines MIP-1α and MIP-1β with the endothelia of the blood-brain barrier. *Neuroscience Letters, 205,* 202–206.

Banks, W.A, Kastin, A.J., & Gutierrez, E.G. (1994). Penetration of interleukin-6 across the murine blood-brain barrier. *Neuroscience Letters, 179,* 53–56.

Banks, W.A, Ortiz, L., Plotkin, S.R., & Kastin, A.J. (1991). Human interleukin (IL) 1α, murine IL-1α and murine IL-β are transported from blood to brain in the mouse by a saturable mechanism. *Journal of Pharmacology and Experimental Therapeutics, 259,* 988–996.

Banks, W.A, Plotkin, S.R., & Kastin, A.J. (1995). Permeability of the blood-brain barrier to soluble cytokine receptors. *Neuroimmunomodulation, 2,* 161–165.

Banks, W.A., Kastin, A.J., & Ehrensing, C.A. (1994). Blood-borne interleukin-1α is transported across the endothelial blood-spinal cord barrier of mice. *Journal of Physiology, 479.2,* 257–264.

Banks, W.A., Kastin, A.J., & Gutierrez, E.G. (1993). Interleukin-1α in blood has direct access to cortical brain cells. *Neuroscience Letters, 163,* 41–44.

Barrera, C.M., Banks, W.A., Fasold, M.B., & Kastin, A.J. (1991). Effects of various reproductive hormones on the penetration of LHRH across the blood-brain barrier. *Pharmacology, Biochemistry and Behavior, 41,* 255–257.

Blomstrand, E., Perrett, D., Parry-Billings, M., & Newsholme, E.A. (1989). Effect of sustained exercise on plasma amino acid concentrations and on 5-hydroxytryptamine metabolism in six different brain regions in the rat. *ACTA Physiologica Scandinavia, 136,* 473–481.

Buchwald, D., Cheney, P.R., Peterson, D.L., Henry, B., Wormsley, S.B., Geiger, A., Ablashi, D.V., Salahuddin, S.Z., Saxinger, C., Biddle, R., Kikinis, R., Jolesz, F.A., Folks, T., Balachandran, N., Peter, J.B., Gallo, R.C., & Komaroff, A.L. (1992). A chronic illness characterized by fatigue, neurologic and immunologic disorders, and active human herpesvirus type 6 infection. *Annals of Internal Medicine, 116,* 103–113.

Buchwald, D. & Komaroff, A.L. (1991). Review of laboratory findings for patients with chronic fatigue syndrome. *Reviews of Infectious Diseases, 13(Suppl 1),* S12–8.

Calogero, A.E., Bernardini, R., Margioris, A.N., Gallucci, W.T., Munson, P.J., Tamarkin, L., Tomai, T.P., Brady, L., Gold, P.W., & Chrousos, G.P. (1989). Effects of serotonergic agonists andantagonists on corticotropin-releasing hormone secretion by explanted rat hypothalami. *Peptides, 10,* 189–200.

Calogero, A.E., Gallucci, W.T., Gold, P.W., & Chrousos, G.P. (1988). Multiple feedback regulatory loops upon rat hypothalamic corticotropin-releasing hormone secretion. *Journal of Clinical Investigation, 82,* 767–774.

Chao, C.C., Janoff, E.N., Hu, S., Thomas, K., Gallagher, M., Tsang, M., & Peterson, P.K. (1991). Altered cytokine release in peripheral blood mononuclear cell cultures from patients with chronic fatigue syndrome. *Cytokine, 3,* 292–298.

Chappell, P.B., Smith, M.A., Kilts, C.D., Bissette, G., Ritchie, J., Anderson, C., & Nemeroff, C.B. (1986). Alterations in corticotropin-releasing factor-like immunoreactivity in discrete rat brain regions after acute and chronic stress. *Journal of Neuroscience, 6,* 2908–2914.

Cleare, A.J., Bearn, J., Allain, T., McGregor, A., Wesseley, S., Murray, R.M., & O'Keane, V. (1995). Contrasting neuroendocrine responses in depression and chronic fatigue syndrome. *Journal of Affective Disorders, 34,* 283–289.

Cotton, P. (1991). Treatment proposed for chronic fatigue syndrome; research continues to compile data on disorder. *Journal of the American Medical Association, 266,* 2667–2668.

Dallman, M.F. (1993). Stress update: adaptation of the hypothalmic-pituitary-adrenal axis to chronic stress. *Trends in Endocrinology and Metabolism, 4,* 62–69.

De Goeij, D.C.E., Binnekade, R., & Tilders, F.J.H. (1992). Chronic stress enhances vasopressin but not corticotropin-releasing factor secretion during hypoglycemia. *American Journal of Physiology, 263,* E394-E399.

DeFreitas, E., Hilliard, B., Cheney, P.R., Bell, D.S., Kiggundi, E., Sankey, D., Wroblewska, Z., Palladino, M., Woodward, J.P., & Koprowski, H. (1991). Retroviral sequences related to human t-lymphotropic virus type II in patients with chronic fatigue immune dysfunction syndrome. *Proceedings of the National Academy of Sciences of the United States of America, 88,* 2922–2926.

Deluca, J., Johnson, S.K., & Natelson, B.H. (1994). Neuropsychiatric status of patients with chronic fatigue syndrome: an overview. *Toxicology and Industrial Health, 10,* 513–522.

Demitrack, M.A., Dale, J.K., Straus, S.E., Laue, L., Listwak, S.J., Kruesi, M.J.P., Chrousos, G.P., & Gold, P.W. (1991). Evidence for impaired activation of the hypothalamic-pituitary-adrenal axis in patients with chronic fatigue syndrome. *Journal of Clinical Endocrinology and Metabolism, 73,* 1224–1234.

Demitrack, M.A., Gold, P.W., Dale, J.K., Krahn, D.D., Kling, M.A., & Straus, S.E. (1992). Plasma and cerebrospinal fluid monoamine metabolism in patients with chronic fatigue syndrome: preliminary findings. *Biological Psychiatry, 32,* 1065–1077.

Demitrack, M.A. (1994). Chronic fatigue syndrome: a disease of the hypothalamic-pituitary-adrenal axis? *Annals of Medicine, 26,* 1–5.

Feldman, S., Conforti, N., & Melamed, E. (1987). Paraventricular nucleus serotonin mediates neurally stimulated adrenocortical secretion. *Brain Research Bulletin, 18,* 165–168.

Flier,J.S.&Underhill,L.H.(1995). The hypothalamic-pituitary-adrenal axis and immune-mediated inflammation. *Seminars in Medicine of the Beth Israel Hospital, Boston, 332,* 1351–1362.

Folks, T.M., Heneine, W., Khan, A., Woods, T., Chapman, L., & Schonberger, L. (1993). Investigation of retroviral involvement in chronic fatigue syndrome. *Ciba Foundation Symposium, 173*, 160–175.

Fukuda, K., Straus, S.E., Hickie, I., Sharpe, M.C., Dobbins, J.G., Komaroff, A., & International Chronic Fatigue Syndrome Study Group, (1994). The chronic fatigue syndrome: a comprehensive approach to its definition and study. *Annals of Internal Medicine, 121*, 953–957.

Fukuda, K. & Gantz, N.M. (1995). Management strategies for chronic fatigue syndrome. *Federal Practitioner*,

Gold, D., Bowden, R., Sixbey, J., Riggs, R., Katon, W.J., Ashley, R., Obrigewitch, R.M., & Corey, L. (1990). Chronic fatigue A prospective clinical and virologic study. *Journal of the American Medical Association, 264*, 48–53.

Goodnick, P.J. & Sandoval, R. (1993). Treatment of chronic fatigue syndrome and related disorders: immunological approaches. In P.J. Goodnick & N.G. Klimas (Eds.). *Chronic Fatigue and Related Immune Deficiency Syndromes* (pp. 109–129). Washington: American Psychiatric Press, Inc.

Gow, J.W., Simpson, K., Schliephake, A., Behan, W.M.H., Morrison, L.J.A., Cavanagh, H., Rethwilm, A., & Behan, P.O. (1992). Search for retrovirus in the chronic fatigue syndrome. *Journal of Clinical Pathology, 45*, 1058–1061.

Gupta, S. & Vayuvegula, B. (1991). A comprehensive immunological analysis in chronic fatigue syndrome. *Scandinavian Journal of Immunology, 33*, 319–327.

Harbuz, M.S., Rees, R.G., Eckland, D., Jessop, D.S., Brewerton, D., & Lightman, S.L. (1992). Paradoxical responses of hypothalamic CRF mRNA and CRF-41 peptide and adenohypophyseal POMC mRNA during chronic inflammatory stress. *Endocrinology, 130*, 1394–1400.

Harbuz, M.S. & Lightman, S.L. (1992). Stress and the hypothalamo-pituitary adrenal axis: acute chronic and immunological activation. *Journal of Endocrinology, 134*, 327–329.

Heneine, W., Woods, T.C., Dinha, S.D., Khan, A.S., Chapman, L.E., Schonberger, L.B., & Folks, T.M. (1994). Lack of evidence for infection with known human and animal retroviruses in patients with chronic fatigue syndrome. *Clinical Infectious Diseases, 18(Suppl 1)*, S121–5.

Hickie, I., Lloyd, A., Wakefield, D., & Parker, G. (1990). The psychiatric status of patients with the chronic fatigue syndrome. *British Journal of Psychiatry, 156*, 534–540.

Hillhouse, E.W. & Milton, N.G.N. (1989). Effect of acetylcholine and 5-hydroxytryptamine on the secretion of corticotrophin-releasing factor-41 and arginine vasopressin from the rat hypothalamas *in vitro*. *Journal of Endocrinology, 122*, 713–718.

Holmes, G.P., Kaplan, J.E., Gantz, N.M., Komaroff, A.L., Schonberger, L.B., Straus, S.E., Jones, J.F., Dubois, R.E., Cunningham-Rundles, C., Pahwa, S., Tosato, G., Zegans, L.S., Purtilo, D.T., Brown, N., Schooley, R.T., & Brus, I. (1988). Chronic fatigue syndrome: a working case definition. *Annals of Internal Medicine, 108,* 387–389.

Hu, S.-B., Lightman, S.L., & Tannahill, L.A. (1992). 5-hdroxytryptamine stimulates corticosteroid-sensitive CRF release from cultured foetal hypothalamic cells. Role of protein kinases. *Brain Research, 574,* 266–270.

Imura, H., Fukata, J.-I., & Mori, T. (1991). Cytokines and endocrine function: an interaction between the immune and neuroendocrine systems. *Clinical Endocrinology, 35,* 107–115.

Jefferies, W.McK. (1994). Mild adrenocortical deficiency, chronic allergies, autoimmune disorders and the chronic fatigue syndrome: a continuation of the cortisone story. *Medical Hypotheses, 42,* 183–189.

Kastin, A.J., Seligson, J., Strimas, J.H., & Chi, D.S. (1991). Failure of metenkephalin to enhance natural killer cell activity. *Immunobiology, 183,* 55–68.

Katon, W.J., Buchwald, D.S., Simon, G.E., Russo, J.E., & Mease, P.J. (1991). Psychiatric illness in patients with chronic fatigue and those with rheumatoid arthritus. *Journal of General Internal Medicine, 6,* 277–285.

Katon, W.J. & Russo, J. (1992). Chronic fatigue syndrome criteria. A critique of the requirement for multiple physical complaints. *Archives of Internal Medicine, 152,* 1604–1609.

Khan, A.S., Heneine, W., Chapman, L.E., Gary, Jr.,H.E., Woods, T.C., Folks, T.M., & Schonberger, L.B. (1993). Assessment of a retrovirus sequence and other possible risk factors for the chronic fatigue syndrome in adults. *Annals of Internal Medicine, 118,* 241–245.

Klimas, N.G., Salvato, F.R., Morgan, R., & Fletcher, M.A. (1990). Immunologic abnormalities in chronic fatigue syndrome. *Journal of Clinical Microbiology, 28,* 1403–1410.

Kruesi, M.J.P., Dale, J., & Straus, S.E. (1989). Psychiatric diagnoses in patients who have chronic fatigue syndrome. *Journal of Clinical Psychiatry, 50,* 53–56.

Landay, A.L., Jessop, C., Lennette, E.T., & Levy, J.A. (1991). Chronic fatigue syndrome: clinical condition associated with immune activation. *The Lancet, 338,* 707–712.

Levy, A.D., Quan, L., Rittenhouse, P.A., & Van de Kar, K.D. (1993). Investigation of the role of 5-HT$_3$ receptors in the secretion of prolactin, ACTH and renin. *Neuroendocrinology, 58,* 65–70.

Levy, J.A. (1994). Part III: Viral studies of chronic fatigue syndrome. *Clinical Infectious Diseases, 18 (Suppl. 1),* S117-S120.

Levy, J.A., Landay, A.L., Jessop, C. & Lennette, E. (1993). Chronic fatigue syndrome: Is it a state of chronic immune activation against on infectious virus? In P.J. Goodnick & N.G. Klimas (Eds.). *Chronic Fatigue and Related Immune Deficiency Syndromes*, (pp. 127–145). Washington: American Psychiatric Press, Inc.

Linde, A., Andersson, B., Svenson, S.B., Ahrne, H., Carlsson, M., Forsberg, P., Hugo, H., Karstorp, A., Lenkei, R., Lindwall, A., Loftenius, A., Sall, C., & Andersson, J. (1992). Serum levels of lymphokines and soluble cellular receptors in primary epstein-barr virus infection and in patients with chronic fatigue syndrome. *Journal of Infectious Diseases*, 165, 994–1000.

Lloyd, A., Gandevia, S., Brockman, A., Hales, J., & Wakefield, D. (1994). Cytokine production and fatigue in patients with chronic fatigue syndrome and healthy control subjects in response to exercise. *Clinical Infectious Diseases*, 18(Suppl 1), S142–6.

Lloyd, A., Hickie, I., Brockman, A., Dwyer, J., & Wakefield, D. (1991). Cytokine levels in serum and cerebrospinal fluid in patients with chronic fatigue syndrome and control subjects. *Journal of Infectious Diseases*, 164, 1023–1024.

MacLeam, G. & Wessely, S. (1994). Professional and popular views of chronic fatigue syndrome. *British Medical Journal*, 308(6931), 776–777.

Maness, L.M., Banks, W.A, Zadina, J.E., & Kastin, A.J. (1995). Selective transport of blood-borne interleukin-1α into the posterior division of the septum of the mouse brain.

Brain Research, 700, 83–88.

Martins, J.M., Kastin, A.J., & Banks, W.A (1996). Unidirectional specific and modulated brain to blood transport of corticotropin-releasing hormone. *Neuroendocrinology*, (in press).

Mawle, A.C., Reyes, M., & Schmid, D.S. (1994). Is chronic fatigue syndrome an infectious disease? *Infectious Agents and Disease*, 2, 333–341.

Meaney, M.J., Mitchell, J.B., Aitken, D.H., Bhatnagar, S., Bodnoff, S.R., Iny, L.J., & Sarrieau, A. (1991). The effects of neonatal handling on the development of the adrenocortical response to stress: implications for neuropathology and cognitive deficits in later life. *Psychoneuroendocrinology*, 16, 85–103.

Mendelson, S.D. & McEwen, B.S. (1992). Autoradiographic analyses of the effects of adrenalectomy and corticosterone on 5-HT_{1A} and 5-HT_{1B} receptors in the dorsal hippocampus and cortex of the rat. *Neuroendocrinology*, 55, 444–450.

Miller, N.A., Carmichael, H.A., Calder, B.D., Behan, P.O., Bell, E.J., McCartney, R.A., & Hall, F.C. (1991). Antibody to coxsackie B virus in diagnosing postviral fatigue syndrome. *British Medical Journal*, 302, 140–143.

Moldofsky, H. (1995). Sleep, neuroimmune and neuroendocrine functions in fibromyalgia and chronic fatigue syndrome. *Advances in Neuroimmunology, 5,* 39–56.

Moldow, R.L., Kastin, A.J., Graf, M., & Fischman, A.J. (1987). Stress mediated changes in hypothalamic corticotropin releasing factorlike immunoreactivity. *Life Sciences, 40,* 413–418.

Morris, R., Sharpe, M., Sharpley, A.L., Cowen, P.J., Hawton, K., & Morris, J. (1993). Abnormalities of sleep in patients with the chronic fatigue syndrome. *British Medical Journal, 306,* 1161–1164.

Newsholme, E.A., Blomstrand, E., Hassmen, P., & Ekblom, B. (1991). Physical and mental fatigue: do changes in plasma amino acids play a role? *Biochemical Society Transactions, 19,* 358–362.

Patarca, R., Fletcher, M.A. & Klimas, N.G. (1993). Immunological correlates of chronic fatigue syndrome. In P.J. Goodnick & N.G. Klimas (Eds.). *Chronic Fatigue and Related Immune Deficiency Syndromes* (pp. 1–21). Washington: American Psychiatric Press, Inc.

Patarca, R., Klimas, N.C., Lugtendorf, S., Antoni, M., & Fletcher, M.A. (1994). Dysregulated expression of tumor necrosis factor in chronic fatigue syndrome: interrelations with cellular sources and patterns of oluble immune mediator expression. *Clinical Infectious Diseases, 18 (Suppl. 1),* S147-S153.

Poteliakhoff, A. (1981). Adrenocortical activity and some clinical findings in acute and chronic fatigue. *Journal of Psychosomatic Research, 25,* 91–95.

Rasmussen, A.K., Nielsen, H., Andersen, V., Barington, T., Bendtzen, K., Hansen, M.B., Nielsen, L., Pedersen, B.K., & Wiik, A. (1994). Chronic fatigue syndrome—a controlled cross sectional study. *Journal of Rheumatology, 21,* 1527–1531.

Reul, J.M.H.M., Stec, I., Wiegars, J.W., Labeur, M.S., Linthorst, A.C.E., & Arzt, E. (1994). Prenatal immune challenge alters the hypothalamic-pituitary-adrenocortical axis in adult rats. *Journal of Clinical Investigation, 93,* 2600–2607.

Sandman, C.A., Barron, J.L., Nackoul, K., Goldstein, J., & Fidler, F. (1993). Memory deficits associated with chronic fatigue immune dysfunction syndrome. *Biological Psychiatry, 33,* 618–623.

Spinedi, E., Salas, M., Chisari, A., Perone, M., Carino, M., & Gaillard, R.C. (1994). Sex differences in the hypothalamo-pituitary-adrenal axis response to inflammatory and neuroendocrine stressors. *Neuroendocrinology, 60,* 609–617.

Sternberg, E.M., Hill, J.M., Chrousos, G.P., Kamilaris, T., Listwak, S.J., Gold, P.W., & Wilder, R.L. (1989). Inflammatory mediator-induced hypothalamic-pituitary-adrenal axis activation is defective in streptococcal cell wall arthritus-susceptible Lewis rats. *Proceedings of the National Academy of Sciences of the United States of America, 86,* 2374–2378.

Straus, S.E., Dale, J.K., Peter, J.B., & Dinarello, C.A. (1989). Circulating lymphokine levels in the chronic fatigue syndrome. *Journal of Infectious Diseases, 160,* 1085–1086.

Straus, S.E., Fritz, S., Dale, J.K., Gould, B., & Strober, W. (1993). Lymphocyte phenotype and function in the chronic fatigue syndrome. *Journal of Clinical Immunology, 13,* 30–40.

Suda, T., Tozawa, F., Ushiyama, T., Sumitoma, T., Yamada, M., & Demura, H. (1990). Interleukin-1 stimulates corticotropin-releasing factor gene expression in rat hypothalamus. *Endocrinology, 126,* 1223–1227.

Swain, M.G., Patchev, V., Vergalla, J., Chrousos, G., & Jones, E.A. (1993). Suppression of hypothalamic-pituitary-adrenal axis responsiveness to stress in a rat model of acute cholestasis. *Journal of Clinical Investigation, 91,* 1903–1908.

Waguespack, P.J., Banks, W.A, & Kastin, A.J. (1994). Interleukin-2 does not cross the blood-brain barrier by a saturable transport system. *Brain Research Bulletin, 34,* 103–109.

Wessely, S., Chalder, T., Hirsch, S., Pawlikowska, T., Wallace, P., & Wright, D.J.M. (1995). Postinfectious fatigue: prospective cohort study in primary care. *The Lancet, 345,* 1333–1338.

Wick, G., Hu, S., Schwarz, S., & Kroemer, G. (1993). Immunoendocrine communications via the hypothalamo-pituitary-adrenal axis in autoimmune diseases. *Endocrine Review, 14,* 539–563.

Wilson, A., Hickie, I., Lloyd, A., & Wakefield, D. (1994). The treatment of chronic fatigue syndrome: science and speculation. *American Journal of Medicine, 95(6),* 544–550.

Zhukov, D.A. (1993). The dexamethasone suppression test in genetically different rats exposed to inescapable and escapable electric shocks. *Psychoneuroendocrinology, 18,* 467–474.

INDEX

DATE DUE

MAY 1 9 1999

RET'D JUL 1 6 2018